Fast Facts:
Bladder Disorders

Second edition

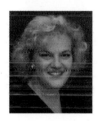

Alex Slack MRCOG

Consultant Urogynaecologist

Maidstone and Tunbridge Wells NHS Trust

Tunbridge Wells, Kent, UK

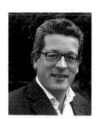

Diane K Newman DNP FAAN BCB-PMD

Co-director, Penn Center for Continence and Pelvic Health

Division of Urology

University of Pennsylvania

Health System, and Senior Research Investigator

University of Pennsylvania

Philadelphia, PA, USA

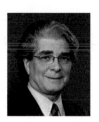

Alan J Wein MD FACS PHD (HON)

Founders Professor of Urology

Perelman School of Medicine

University of Pennsylvania, and

Chief of Urology

Penn Medicine/University of Pennsylvania Health System

Perelman Center for Advanced Medicine

Philadelphia, PA, USA

Declaration of Independence
This book is as balanced and as practical as we can make it.
Ideas for improvement are always welcome: feedback@fastfacts.com

 HEALTH PRESS

Fast Facts: Bladder Disorders
First published 2008
Second edition August 2011

Health Press Limited, Elizabeth House, Queen Street, Abingdon,
Oxford OX14 3LN, UK
Tel: +44 (0)1235 523233
Fax: +44 (0)1235 523238

Book orders can be placed by telephone or via the website.
For regional distributors or to order via the website, please go to:
www.fastfacts.com
For telephone orders, please call +44 (0)1752 202301 (UK, Europe and Asia–
Pacific), 1 800 247 6553 (USA, toll free) or +1 419 281 1802 (Americas).

Fast Facts is a trademark of Health Press Limited.

A CIP record for this title is available from the British Library.

ISBN 978-1-905832-96-5

Slack A (Alex)
Fast Facts: Bladder Disorders/
Alex Slack, Diane K Newman, Alan J Wein

Medical illustrations by Dee McLean, London, UK.
Typesetting and page layout by Zed, Oxford, UK.
Printed by Latimer Trend and Company Ltd, Plymouth UK.

Text printed on biodegradable and recyclable paper
manufactured using elemental chlorine free (ECF) wood pulp
from well-managed forests.

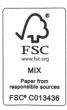

FSC
www.fsc.org
MIX
Paper from
responsible sources
FSC® C013436

Introduction

'Bladder disorders' is an inclusive term that encompasses a number of lower urinary tract dysfunctions and abnormalities, which affect a significant number of individuals. These disorders can have a substantial negative effect on quality of life, and some can cause considerable morbidity and even mortality.

This book was written with the non-specialist healthcare professional in mind, to provide the 'fundamentals' related to a number of these disorders – enough to recognize the symptoms and signs, understand the basic pathophysiology and institute screening and assessment and, where appropriate, initial treatment.

We intended the content to be based on evidence and expert opinion as much as possible, balanced where opinions are not unanimous and, above all, practical and useful for clinical practice. This edition, the second, incorporates the significant agreed upon advancements in the field and further elaborates on topics that some readers considered to be under-represented in the first edition. Ideas for further improvements are welcome.

1 Anatomy and function of the urinary system

Anatomy

A complete description of the anatomy of the urinary system is beyond the scope of this book and is of limited interest to the general healthcare professional. However, particular aspects of the anatomy and function of the urinary tract are relevant to understanding bladder disorders and should be familiar to anyone working in the field. The relevant anatomy of the urinary system is shown in Figure 1.1.

The term 'internal sphincter' is often used and refers to the smooth muscle of the bladder neck and proximal urethra. Control of the internal sphincter is involuntary. The term 'external sphincter' or 'external urethral sphincter' refers to the striated muscle that surrounds the proximal urethra and is under voluntary control. Some striated muscle also forms part of the urethra for a variable distance from the bladder neck. The entire striated sphincter complex is often referred to as the 'rhabdosphincter'.

Function

Continence is maintained by a complex interaction between the bladder, the urethra, the pelvic floor muscles, the endopelvic fascia and the nervous system. The bladder operates as a low-pressure high-volume system, pressure increasing slowly and steadily as the bladder fills, normally at a rate of 0.5–5 mL/minute. It can usually hold 500–600 mL urine. A first need to void is felt when the bladder contains 250–300 mL. Continence is maintained as long as the urethral pressure exceeds the bladder pressure.

During normal voiding, voluntary relaxation of the striated musculature in and around the urethra precedes contraction of the detrusor (bladder) muscle. The bladder neck and proximal urethra (often referred to as the 'bladder outlet') become funnel shaped. This relaxation/contraction combination reduces outflow resistance and increases intravesical (in the bladder) pressure, causing the bladder to be emptied forcibly.

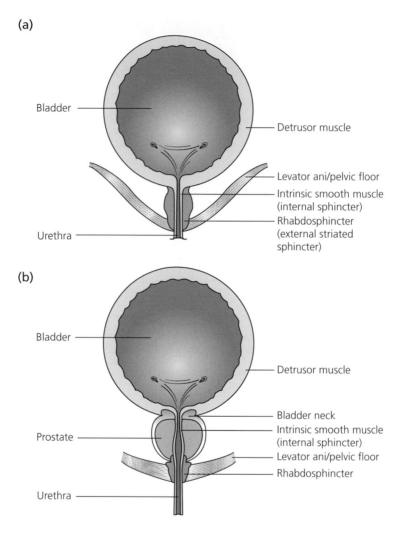

Figure 1.1 Key anatomic features of (a) female and (b) male lower urinary systems.

Urine storage and voiding are controlled by reflex centers in the spinal cord and the micturition center in the midbrain. Both the autonomic and somatic nervous systems are involved. The innervation of the bladder is shown in Figure 1.2. The main neurological pathways that affect bladder contraction are parasympathetic. The sacral reflex center is situated in S2 to S4, and the pelvic nerve and its branches

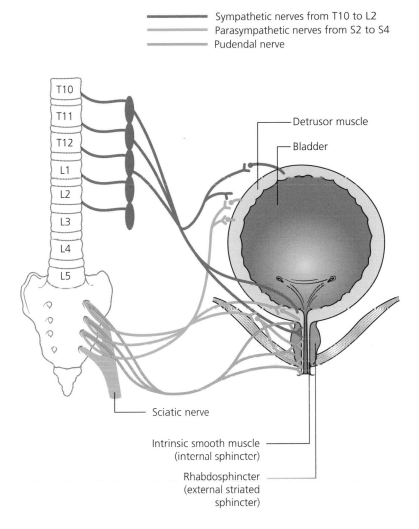

Figure 1.2 Innervation of the bladder.

lead from here to the detrusor muscle. Excitation of these nerves stimulates the release primarily of acetylcholine, which acts on muscarinic receptors to cause detrusor contraction.

During normal bladder filling, there is no excitatory input from the micturition center in the brain to the sacral micturition center or from the sacral micturition center to the pelvic nerves. The detrusor

TABLE 1.1

Requirements for bladder filling/urine storage and voiding

Bladder filling/urine storage requires:

- accommodation of an increasing volume of urine at low intravesical pressure (normal compliance) and with normal sensations
- a bladder outlet that is closed at rest and remains closed during increases in intra-abdominal pressure
- absence of involuntary bladder contractions (detrusor overactivity)

Bladder emptying/voiding requires:

- a coordinated contraction of the bladder smooth musculature of adequate magnitude and duration
- a concomitant lowering of resistance at the level of the smooth and striated sphincter (bladder outlet)
- absence of anatomic (as opposed to functional) obstruction

(bladder) is quiescent. There is a gradual increase in the tone of the external sphincter (striated muscle), mediated through impulses via the pudendal nerve.

Voiding depends on coordinated excitation of the sacral parasympathetic nerves and simultaneous opening of the bladder outlet (involuntary) and relaxation of the external urethral sphincter (voluntary); continence requires the converse (Table 1.1). Storage and voluntary emptying of the bladder are also influenced by psychological and sociocultural factors. Adults are trained to void in a socially acceptable place and women may not want or like to void in any other place than their homes because of concern about unsafe or unsanitary toilet facilities. Using a toilet away from home can cause psychological stress, suppression of the desire to void and infrequent voiding. Voiding position and posture (e.g. squatting or sitting) used by women to empty the bladder differs by cultures or by health status. Negative perceptions of the physical environment of toilets can alter toileting stance or suppress the desire to void.

Key points – anatomy and function of the urinary system

- The bladder operates as a low-pressure high-volume system.
- Urine storage and voiding are controlled by reflex centers in the spinal cord, the micturition center in the midbrain and the somatic and parasympathetic nervous systems.
- Voiding requires a coordinated contraction of the detrusor (bladder smooth musculature), simultaneous opening of the bladder outlet (involuntary) and relaxation of the external urethral sphincter (voluntary). Continence requires the converse.

Key references

Ashton-Miller JA, DeLancey JO. Functional anatomy of the female pelvic floor. *Ann NY Acad Sci* 2007;1101:266–96.

Brooks JD. Anatomy of the lower urinary tract and male genitalia. In: Wein AJ, Kavoussi LR, Novick AC et al., eds. *Campbell-Walsh Urology*, 9th edn. Philadelphia: Saunders/ Elsevier, 2007:38–77.

Keane DP, O'Sullivan S. Urinary incontinence: anatomy, physiology and pathophysiology. *Baillieres Best Pract Res Clin Obstet Gynaecol* 2000;14:207–26.

Newman DK, Wein AJ. *Managing and Treating Urinary Incontinence*, 2nd edn. Baltimore: Health Professions Press, 2009:61–84.

Wang K, Palmer MH. Women's toileting behaviour related to urinary elimination: concept analysis. *J Adv Nurs* 2010;66:1874–84.

Wein AJ, Moy ML. Voiding function, dysfunction and urinary incontinence. In: Hanno P, Wein AJ, Malkowicz SB, eds. *Penn Clinical Manual of Urology*. Philadelphia: Saunders/Elsevier, 2007:341–478.

History

Urologic symptoms are clearly a key aspect in the diagnosis of urinary disorders, but may not be reliable when used alone; as many have stated, the bladder may be an unreliable witness. The onset of urinary symptoms, their duration and severity, and the time(s) when they occur, should be recorded. Symptoms can be divided into filling/storage, voiding/emptying and postmicturition.

Filling symptoms

Frequency is the complaint of voiding too often by day and is usually defined as more than eight voids per 24 hours. Increased daytime frequency can occur with a normal bladder capacity where there is excessive fluid intake, or where the bladder capacity is affected by detrusor overactivity, impaired bladder compliance (compliance refers to the tonic change in bladder pressure during filling – usually, bladder compliance is normal if there is little or no change in detrusor pressure during filling) or increased bladder sensation (hypersensitivity). The causes of daytime frequency are shown in Table 2.1.

Nocturia is the complaint of waking to void one or more times during the night. It may occur for the same reasons as daytime frequency, but may also occur in association with congestive heart failure (causing nocturnal polyuria) or because the normal circadian rhythm of antidiuretic hormone (ADH; desmopressin) secretion becomes reversed.

Urgency is a sudden compelling desire to void that is difficult to defer. Urgency implies detrusor overactivity, but can also occur if there is an underlying bladder inflammatory disorder.

Storage symptoms

Stress (or effort-related) incontinence is the involuntary loss of urine during physical exertion. This occurs without any contraction of the

TABLE 2.1

Causes of daytime urinary frequency

- Detrusor overactivity (urodynamic finding)
- Impaired bladder compliance (urodynamic finding)
- Increased bladder sensation
- Overactive bladder (symptom syndrome)
- Excessive fluid intake
- Medication that causes diuresis (e.g. diuretic)
- Diabetes mellitus
- Caffeine intake (in susceptible individuals)
- Prophylactic or 'defensive' voiding (to avoid urgency or urgency incontinence)

detrusor and may be associated with a number of physical activities, including laughing, coughing, sneezing, running, jumping, aerobics and sexual activity. Urine loss is usually in small amounts (drops, squirts) and may not be a daily event. It is caused by failure of the bladder outlet to remain closed and thereby maintain continence when intra-abdominal pressure is raised.

Urgency (previously called urge) incontinence is the involuntary leakage of urine accompanied, or immediately preceded, by urgency. Urgency incontinence can take the form of frequent small losses between voids or large urine losses from sudden complete bladder emptying. It can occur several times a day or week. It is caused by involuntary detrusor contractions during bladder filling/urine storage.

Nocturnal enuresis is the loss of urine during sleep. When taking a history, it is important to inquire about childhood nocturnal enuresis (bed-wetting), as delayed bladder control in childhood is often associated with detrusor overactivity in adulthood.

Continuous incontinence tends to be associated with urinary tract fistulas or with chronic urinary retention with so-called overflow incontinence. Urinary tract fistulas are usually iatrogenic in developed countries, but are commonly associated with unsupervised childbirth in developing countries. Chronic retention is most common in men with obstruction secondary to prostate enlargement or in women with severe pelvic organ prolapse (POP), such as vaginal vault prolapse.

Mixed incontinence is the coexistence of stress incontinence with urgency incontinence or urge symptoms.

Pressure (bladder, suprapubic) is the sensation that the bladder is full and the urge to void will occur shortly. Its causes include incomplete bladder emptying. Discomfort that is relieved by voiding may indicate interstitial cystitis or bladder pain syndrome.

Voiding/emptying symptoms

With the exception of postmicturition dribble, all of the symptoms described below can be associated with bladder outlet obstruction, a poorly contracting detrusor or loss of coordination between detrusor contractility and relaxation of the external urethral sphincter, termed detrusor–sphincter dyssynergia (DSD). These symptoms are more often seen in men than in women.

Hesitancy is described as difficulty in initiating micturition, resulting in a delay in the onset of voiding when the individual is ready to pass urine.

Intermittent stream or intermittency describes urine flow that stops and starts once or more during micturition.

Slow stream is the perception of a reduced urine flow, usually compared with previous performance or with the flow of others.

Terminal dribble describes a prolonged final part of micturition, when the flow slows to a trickle.

Incomplete emptying is a self-explanatory term for a feeling experienced by an individual after passing urine.

Postmicturition dribble refers to the leakage of urine after micturition. Approximately 80% of men experience this symptom at some time, and it can present at any age. The symptom arises from the leakage of a few drops of urine that are pooled in the bulbar urethra after micturition has been completed and that drain under gravity a few moments later. Postmicturition dribble is seldom associated with clinical abnormalities, and can be avoided by waiting until the remaining urine has been passed or by milking the urethra at the end of micturition (Figure 2.1). Urethral stricture or diverticulum may be rare causes of this condition. If voiding dysfunction is present, uroflowmetry should be the first investigation (see page 25).

Physical examination
All patients presenting with bladder symptoms should undergo a full physical examination, including neurological examination.

Neurological examination. Neurological conditions that are associated with bladder problems (such as multiple sclerosis, stroke, Parkinson's disease or spinal injury) are usually obvious when the patient first presents.

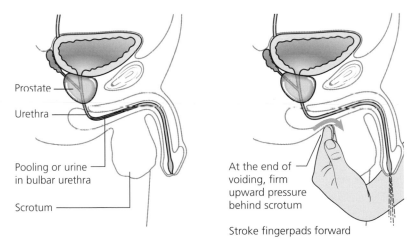

Prostate

Urethra

Pooling or urine in bulbar urethra

Scrotum

At the end of voiding, firm upward pressure behind scrotum

Stroke fingerpads forward

Figure 2.1 Post-void dribble technique to help expel remaining urine. At the end of voiding, firm upward pressure is applied behind the scrotum and fingers stroke forward. Redrawn with permission from Diane K Newman.

If a neurological cause is suspected, it is important to pay particular attention to sacral neuronal pathways. The gait, abduction and dorsiflexion of the toes (S3) should be assessed, as should sensory innervation of the perineum (L1–L2), sole and lateral aspect of the foot (S1) and posterior aspect of the thigh (S2). Perineal (S3) and cutaneous reflexes (bulbocavernosus and anal reflexes) should also be tested.

Abdominal examination. Scars from previous surgery should be noted. Increased abdominal striae may be found in association with other markers of abnormal collagen metabolism, and are more common in women with POP and stress incontinence.

An attempt to palpate the kidneys should be made. Abdominal examination or suprapubic percussion may identify a distended bladder (if more than 300 mL in bladder) or a pelvic mass that is compressing the bladder.

Genital examination is essential in both women and men.

Women. The urethral meatus, skin of the vulva and perineum should be examined, and any atrophic vaginitis identified. Excoriation and maceration of the vulva may occur with constant wetness and may cause secondary infections.

Speculum examination will enable assessment of the vaginal walls to identify atrophy, urethral caruncle or POP (cystocele, rectocele, uterine or vaginal vault prolapse). Pelvic masses may also be identified. The woman should be asked to cough and strain in an attempt to demonstrate stress incontinence. Ideally, this should be done with a full bladder. It may be necessary to examine the woman whilst she stands with one foot on a stool, in order to detect POP or stress incontinence.

The strength of the pelvic floor muscles (PFM) should be assessed and can be quantified using a validated grading system such as the Oxford 1–5 scale. Factors to be assessed include strength, duration and repeatability of contractions, and displacement of the pelvic floor. Low-tone pelvic floor dysfunction refers to the examination findings of an impaired ability to isolate and contract the pelvic floor musculature in the presence of weak and atrophic musculature and is seen in women with POP, urinary or fecal incontinence, and vaginal weakness. High-tone pelvic floor dysfunction refers to the clinical condition of hypertonic spastic PFM with resultant impairment of muscle isolation, contraction and relaxation and is seen in women with interstitial cystitis/bladder pain syndrome, voiding dysfunction, overactive bladder, pelvic pain and sexual dysfunction with dyspareunia.

Men. The appearance of the external urethral meatus and prepuce may be a guide to distal urethral causes of voiding difficulties or postmicturition dribble that the patient may describe as urinary incontinence (i.e. strictures).

Digital rectal examination (see Figure 5.1, page 66) should include palpation of the prostate to assess size, symmetry and consistency of the gland, its position in relation to the rectum and pelvic side wall and the presence of nodularity or induration. Symptoms of bladder overactivity can be caused by locally advanced prostate cancer or an enlarged prostate.

Rectal masses are obviously abnormal and require prompt referral. The status of the anal sphincter musculature should be noted by determining strength and tone.

Further investigations

Further investigation is usually necessary to confirm the cause of bladder symptoms. The investigations undertaken will depend to some extent on the facilities available.

Psychological and cognitive assessment. The patient should be assessed for clinical depression, which can compromise the success of behavioral and surgical treatments. A mini mental-state examination or clock-drawing test can be used if cognitive impairment is suspected, as incontinence can be related to memory changes.

Functional and environment assessment. In elderly patients, an assessment of functional abilities should focus on self-care tasks or activities of daily living (ADL) (ability to ambulate, disrobe). Mobility problems (e.g. inability to access the toilet, history of falls) are stronger predictors for developing urinary incontinence than cognitive impairment. Environmental assessment should include identifying the location of the toilet

Quality of life. There are a number of ways to assess the impact of incontinence symptoms on a patient's quality of life. However, the only valid way to measure the patient's perception of their symptoms is through the use of psychometrically robust self-completion questionnaires, such as the International Continence Society's International Consultation on Incontinence modular questionnaire (ICIQ; Figure 2.2) A wide variety of questionnaires were assessed by the Continence Society the questionnaires recommended for the assessment of quality of life for patients with urinary incontinence alone or in the presence of lower urinary tract symptoms are listed in Table 2.2.

Frequency/volume bladder record. Use of a bladder record or diary is a simple and practical method to obtain information on a patient's normal voiding pattern, including frequency and amount of micturition and episodes of leakage, in addition to the time and volume of fluid ingested. The patient records the times and volumes of all voids over a specific time period, which should be at least 24 hours so that both day and night are included. Episodes of urinary incontinence are recorded and whether they are associated with, for example, urgency, straining or coughing. Eliciting an estimate of the volume of leakage during incontinence episodes is helpful. The following descriptions of urine leakage can be used.

- Small volume (< 30 mL) – enough to make underwear wet if no protective pad is worn.
- Moderate volume (31–100 mL) – enough to wet or soak underwear and leak down the legs if no protective pad is worn.
- Large volume (101+ mL) – soaks through clothing and onto floor or furniture and usually is the entire bladder volume.

Objective information is obtained not only on daytime frequency and nocturia, but also on the normal functional bladder capacity, mean voided volume, total voided volumes and diurnal distribution of micturition.

☐☐ ☐☐ ☐☐☐ ICIQ-UI Short Form ☐☐ ☐☐ ☐☐

Initial number   **CONFIDENTIAL** DAY MONTH YEAR

               Today's date

Many people leak urine some of the time. We are trying to find out how many people leak urine, and how much this bothers them. We would be grateful if you could answer the following questions, thinking about how you have been, on average, over the PAST FOUR WEEKS.

1 Please write in your date of birth: ☐☐ ☐☐ ☐☐

               DAY MONTH YEAR

2 Are you *(tick one)*:   Female ☐ Male ☐

---

3 How often do you leak urine? *(Tick one box)*

            never ☐ 0

    about once a week or less often ☐ 1

     two or three times a week ☐ 2

       about once a day ☐ 3

      several times a day ☐ 4

        all the time ☐ 5

---

4 We would like to know how much urine <u>you think</u> leaks.
How much urine do you <u>usually</u> leak (whether you wear protection or not)?
(Tick one box)

           none ☐ 0

      a small amount ☐ 2

    a moderate amount ☐ 4

     a large amount ☐ 6

---

5 Overall, how much does leaking urine interfere with your everyday life?
Please ring a number between 0 (not at all) and 10 (a great deal)

    0 1 2 3 4 5 6 7 8 9 **10**
   not at all   a great deal

      ICIQ score: sum scores 3+4+5 ☐ ☐

---

6 When does urine leak? *(Please tick all that apply to you)*

        never – urine does not leak ☐

     leaks before you can get to the toilet ☐

      leaks when you cough or sneeze ☐

        leaks when you are asleep ☐

  leaks when you are physically active/exercising ☐

leaks when you have finished urinating and are dressed ☐

       leaks for no obvious reason ☐

         leaks all the time ☐

Thank you very much for answering these questions.

Figure 2.2 This short-form international consultation on incontinence modular questionnaire (ICIQ) is one of a number of questionnaires that have been validated to assess a patient's perception of their symptoms. Reproduced with permission of the ICIQ Group. See www.iciq.net for further information.

TABLE 2.2

Questionnaires recommended by the International Continence Society for assessing quality of life in patients with urinary incontinence

Men and women	International consultation on incontinence modular questionnaire (ICIQ-UI short form; see Figure 2.2)
Women	ICIQ-FLUTS, formerly known as the Bristol female lower urinary tract symptoms short-form questionnaire
	Stress and urge incontinence quality-of-life questionnaire (SUIQQ)
Men	ICIQ-MLUTS, formerly known as the International Continence Society male short-form questionnaire

Abnormalities that may be demonstrated on a frequency/volume bladder record include:

- regular voiding of small quantities of urine, which is associated with filling abnormalities or may be a result of defensive voiding (voiding to ensure an empty bladder so as to decrease the chance of urine leakage)
- nocturia and nocturnal polyuria (passing more than one-third of the 24-hour output during normal sleeping hours)
- fluid restriction
- excessive fluid intake (through habit or on medical advice)
- polyuria (an excessive volume of urination, which in an adult would be more than 2500 mL/day)
- urinary incontinence and the associated circumstances (i.e. urgency, effort, unaware)
- type and number of absorbent pads used.

The frequency/volume bladder record is also useful for assessing and monitoring treatment, and to demonstrate the benefits of treatment to a patient. An example of a completed record is shown in Figure 2.3.

Urinalysis and culture. Dipstick urinalysis is used to detect hematuria, glycosuria, pyuria and bacteriuria. It should be carried out for all patients presenting with urinary incontinence to exclude the possibility

FREQUENCY/VOLUME BLADDER DIARY

Time	Amount voided (ounces or ccs)	Urine leakage	Reason for urine leakage or voiding (urgency, coughing, bending)	Amount and type of fluid intake
1:30 am	5 oz		Woke up, went to toilet	2 oz water
4 am	6 oz			
6:30 am	5 oz	✓	Urgency, rushing to toilet	3 oz water
7 am				8 oz coffee, 6 oz juice
7:30 am	4 oz		Washing face, urgency	
9:30 am				6 oz coffee
11:30 am	8 oz	✓	Urgency	4 oz water
12:15 pm	4oz		Slight urgency	
12:30 pm				7 oz water, 8 oz diet soda
1 pm	7 oz			
3:15 pm	5 oz		Strong urge	4 oz red bull
6 pm	6 oz	✓		
7 pm				4 oz water, 8 oz diet soda, 4 oz glass wine
8:15 pm	7 oz		Urgency	
10:30 pm	4 oz			

Circle the product
you are using

Number of products
used __3__

Pantiliners

Pads

Underwear

Brief or Diaper

Analysis : 66 yo female with OAB symptoms of urgency with urgency incontinence and frequency which occurs 11 times (nocturia x 3). Fluid intake of 64 ozs with a large caffeinated beverage intake. Patient voids frequently (61 ozs) and mostly in small amounts.

Figure 2.3 The frequency/volume bladder record (bladder diary) is a simple method of highlighting abnormal fluid intake and increased frequency of micturition. The diary shown indicates: (1) frequent voiding of small volumes of urine, indicative of a filling disorder such as overactive bladder; (2) fairly large intake of bladder irritant beverages (e.g. liquids containing caffeine); (3) urine leakage preceded by urgency; (4) less than one-third of the 24-hour urine output being passed during sleeping hours (more than one-third volume would be indicative of nocturnal polyuria (see pages 96–8); (5) use of three perineal pads per day which may indicate a moderate to severe amount of urine leakage but this should be clarified with the patient.

of infection, inflammation, urinary tract malignancy and diabetes. A positive dipstick test should be followed up by formal urine microscopy and culture to detect a urinary tract infection (UTI) before treatment and to allow antibiotic sensitivity to be evaluated. The presence of hematuria or red blood cells on microscopy should be investigated further with urine cytology, an imaging study of the upper tracts (kidneys and ureters) and endoscopic examination of the bladder and urethra to rule out malignancy, especially in a patient over 50 years of age with symptoms of bladder irritation. The investigation and management of hematuria are described in detail in Chapter 6.

Imaging

Radiography. A preliminary plain abdominal radiograph can be performed in patients with suspected renal tract calculi or soft tissue masses.

Ultrasonography has become the first-line method for detecting abnormalities of the kidneys, including scarring, calculi, dilatation and tumors. Ultrasound can also be used to detect increased bladder-wall thickness (which suggests outlet obstruction and/or detrusor overactivity) and to look for bladder calculi; portable ultrasound devices or 'bladder scanners' can be used to measure postvoid urine volumes.

Intravenous urography has largely been superseded by ultrasound for initial investigation of microscopic hematuria but may be appropriate if ultrasonography suggests obstruction or leakage from a fistula.

CT urography has become the investigation of choice if ultrasonography is not diagnostic or gross hematuria is present. It has a higher sensitivity for small calculi and early neoplasms.

Urodynamic studies

These include tests that generate quantitative data relevant to events in the bladder and bladder outlet during the filling/storage and emptying/voiding phases of micturition.

Many clinicians request urodynamic investigation for any patient, especially a woman, who complains of lower urinary tract symptoms; however, the clinician may have little appreciation of the clinical indications, what the test involves and its limitations. Urodynamic investigation is safe, but men in particular may experience some discomfort related to catheterization, which can last for up to 24 hours after the test. The incidence of culture-proven UTI following urodynamic testing is approximately 1%; prophylactic antibiotics should therefore be considered for patients who may be at risk (e.g. immunosuppression or prosthesis implanted within last 2 years).

Indications. Urodynamic investigation may be indicated in the following cases:
- treatment failure
- complex mixed lower urinary tract symptoms
- before incontinence surgery
- symptoms suggesting detrusor overactivity
- voiding symptoms
- women with POP
- urinary retention
- neurogenic disease.

Complex mixed lower urinary tract symptoms or treatment failure. Some patients present with such a complicated history that it is impossible to make any judgment as to the cause of their symptoms. Empirical treatment is therefore not possible. The patient should undergo urodynamic investigation so that appropriate treatment can be offered.

Before incontinence surgery. In our opinion, urodynamic information is essential if surgery to treat incontinence, especially stress incontinence, is contemplated. There is, however, some debate as to the need for urodynamic investigation before incontinence surgery. The UK's National Institute for Health and Clinical Excellence (NICE) has issued guidelines stating that preoperative urodynamic studies are not necessary for patients undergoing a primary procedure and whose symptoms and examination findings suggest simple stress incontinence. We disagree with this recommendation, as it has been

23

claimed that surgery carried out on the basis of symptoms alone is inappropriate in up to 25% of cases. Furthermore, surgery for stress incontinence can lead to voiding dysfunction and de novo detrusor overactivity (the urodynamic term describing involuntary bladder contraction), or may exacerbate pre-existing symptoms, so it is important to perform a preoperative assessment.

Symptoms suggesting detrusor overactivity. Most patients with symptoms suggestive of detrusor overactivity can be treated empirically. This assumes that other obvious causes for the symptoms (e.g. urinary infection) have been excluded and that neither hematuria (blood in the urine) nor significant bladder, urethral or pelvic pain is present. Urodynamic investigation is appropriate if symptoms of detrusor overactivity are unresponsive to drug and/or behavioral therapy and if the diagnosis is essential, either to avoid unnecessary continuation of drugs or to exclude other pathology. It is important to understand that a urodynamic study provides only an artificial 10–20-minute 'snapshot' and does not always replicate real-life events. Thus, a patient with symptoms of detrusor overactivity may have a normal urodynamic study. Some of these patients will have detrusor overactivity that has been missed, and a trial of drug and/or behavioral therapy is entirely appropriate.

Voiding symptoms and urinary retention are more common in men than women, reflecting a higher incidence of bladder outlet obstruction; however, voiding symptoms do occur in women, especially in association with POP or poor detrusor contractility. The initial investigation should be measurement of free urinary flow and postvoid residual volume. If abnormal emptying is confirmed, full urodynamic assessment is required to differentiate between detrusor hypocontractility and outlet obstruction or both.

Pelvic Organ Prolapse. Urodynamic investigations can be useful prior to undertaking surgery for POP as it is common for this to coexist with urinary incontinence. Treatment of POP can also unmask urinary incontinence that was being concealed by urethral kinking. In this situation it is common to carry out urodynamic investigations with a temporary ring pessary in place.

Neuropathic bladder. Patients with neurological disease and lower urinary tract symptoms are at risk of neurogenic detrusor overactivity, low compliance and DSD. The main concern is the potential for upper urinary tract damage resulting from increased detrusor/intravesical pressure, which can lead to dilatation of the ureters and renal impairment. A simultaneous investigation of the renal tract anatomy and function may be valuable in these patients (videocystourethrography with concurrent urodynamic investigation).

Uroflowmetry is a simple test in which the patient voids in privacy into a commode that incorporates a urinary flowmeter that measures urine flow over time (Figure 2.4). A voided volume of at least 150 mL is desirable for the flow rate to be interpreted accurately. Normal findings are:
- total voided volume greater than 200 mL
- volume passed over a period of 15–20 seconds
- maximum flow rate above 20 mL/second
- smooth crescendo parabolic curve.

It should be recognized that most 'normal' data relate to uroflowmetry in patients younger than 55 years of age; thus, flow rate should be interpreted with consideration for the minimum acceptable flow for given sex and age groups.

Subsequent measurement of the postvoid residual volume by bladder scanning or catheterization gives further information about bladder emptying.

Cystometry records bladder pressure during filling and voiding, with the aim of explaining a clinical problem in pathophysiological terms. The bladder is filled with a saline-like solution at room temperature via a small-bore urethral catheter, alongside which is passed a fine pressure transducer. The pressure in the rectum is recorded simultaneously to differentiate rises in intravesical pressure secondary to increases in abdominal pressure (e.g. coughing, straining, talking and changing position) from those due to detrusor contractions. Table 2.3 lists the measurements required during filling cystometry. Figure 2.5 shows some typical traces.

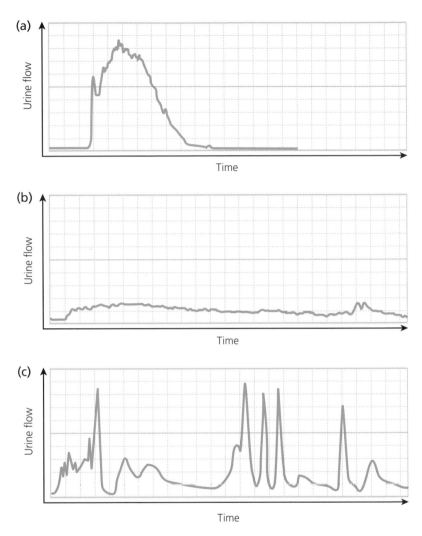

Figure 2.4 Measurement of urine flow rate can indicate a number of abnormalities. (a) Normal voiding. (b) Reduced flow in a man with prostate outlet obstruction. (c) Intermittent increases in flow in a patient straining to void.

Filling cystometry is unphysiological in that the bladder is normally filled at a very slow rate without any change in pressure, and higher filling rates may produce significant artifacts, particularly in patients with neurological problems. Filling rates are classified as follows:

TABLE 2.3

Measurements required during filling cystometry

Intravesical pressure	Usually measured manometrically with a fluid-filled urethral catheter
Intra-abdominal pressure	Measured manometrically with a fluid-filled rectal catheter
Detrusor pressure	Total intravesical pressure minus intra-abdominal pressure
Volume infused	Equates to the bladder volume
Urine flow rate	Measured by mechanical flowmeter

- fast: above 100 mL/minute
- medium: 10–100 mL/min
- slow: less than 10 mL/min.

A filling rate of 50–60 mL/min during conventional filling cystometry appears to be a good compromise, allowing practical filling times with a low incidence of artifacts.

The following can be evaluated during filling cystometry.

- Capacity – the volume infused during filling is measured, and hence the bladder volume is calculated.
- Sensation – the patient is asked to comment on bladder sensation during filling.
- First sensation of bladder filling – this is the feeling that the patient has when he or she first becomes aware of bladder filling during filling cystometry, usually at about half capacity (150–200 mL).
- First desire to void – this is the feeling that leads the patient to pass urine at the next convenient moment, although voiding can be delayed if necessary; commonly at 75% of capacity.
- Strong desire to void – this is a persistent desire to void but without fear of leakage, felt at capacity.
- Urgency – this is a sudden compelling desire to void, described particularly by patients with detrusor overactivity or inflammatory bladder conditions.

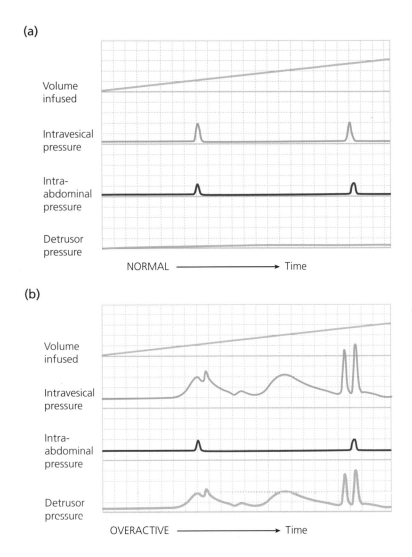

Figure 2.5 Examples of traces obtained from cystometry. (a) A normal trace. (b) Detrusor overactivity. The terms are described in Table 2.3.

- Maximum cystometric capacity – this is the volume at which the patient feels unable to delay micturition (though the test is usually stopped before this).
- Detrusor function – abnormal detrusor contractions during bladder filling are noted; detrusor contractility during voiding can be

assessed by recording the detrusor pressure in the voiding phase.

- Compliance – this indicates the change in volume for a change in pressure and is expressed in mL/cmH_2O. Little or no pressure change occurs during normal filling in a patient with normal compliance. Compliance may be reduced if bladder pathology is present or in patients with neurological disease or injury.
- Urethral function – an incompetent urethral closure mechanism is defined as one that allows leakage of urine in the absence of a detrusor contraction. Stress incontinence can be demonstrated by asking the patient to cough during the filling phase. If urine loss is noted, the subtracted detrusor pressure trace should be checked to ensure that there is no associated detrusor contraction. If stress incontinence has not been demonstrated once the functional bladder capacity is reached, the filling catheter can be removed, leaving a pressure-recording catheter or transducer in place, and the patient is asked to undertake a variety of provocative maneuvers, such as coughing, squatting, heel bouncing and jumping.

Voiding cystometry (pressure–flow study). When filling cystometry has been completed, the filling line is removed as described above, and the patient is asked to void with the bladder and abdominal pressure transducers still in place. The urinary flow rate and detrusor pressure are recorded. A normal man voids with a detrusor pressure of $20–40$ cmH_2O and a normal woman with a considerably lower pressure of $0–25$ cmH_2O. Measurement of detrusor pressure gives an indication of the contractility of the bladder and, when combined with the urinary flow rate, the outflow resistance: high pressures and low flow rates indicate outlet obstruction.

Videourodynamic investigation combines cystometry with simultaneous radiological screening of the bladder and urethra. A radiopaque contrast medium is used instead of saline. Videourodynamic investigation provides information about the appearance of the bladder, urethra and sphincters, and will identify reflux into the ureters. It may be more useful than cystometry alone in the assessment of complex cases. It is especially useful to identify the site of obstruction in an individual with high pressure–low flow and to differentiate low pressure–low flow from outlet obstruction.

Diagnostic cystourethroscopy can be carried out using either a rigid or a flexible cystoscope, with or without anesthesia. Water is the preferred distension medium used during cystoscopy. An angled (flexible) cystoscope (30 or 70 degrees) is normally required to visualize the whole of the bladder. Comment should be made on the appearance of the urethra, trigone, bladder mucosa and ureteric orifices. If bladder filling symptoms are present, the volume of fluid infused should be noted.

Diagnostic cystourethroscopy is indicated in cases of recurrent UTI, hematuria, bladder pain and suspected bladder injury. It is also used intraoperatively when carrying out continence procedures and when inserting suprapubic catheters.

Key points – assessment

- Lower urinary tract symptoms are key in the diagnosis of bladder disorders: onset, duration and severity should be recorded.
- Urinary symptoms can relate to filling (frequency, nocturia, urgency), storage (stress incontinence, urgency incontinence, nocturnal enuresis) or voiding/emptying (hesitancy, intermittent stream, slow stream, terminal dribble, incomplete emptying).
- Physical examination is essential, and may include neurological examination, abdominal examination and examination of the genitals.
- Other assessments include cognitive and mobility evaluation, especially in the elderly.
- The effect of symptoms on quality of life can be assessed using self-completion questionnaires.
- A frequency/volume bladder record (bladder diary) is a simple and practical method to record voiding and fluid intake.
- Dipstick urinalysis is essential for all patients with urinary incontinence, bladder or urethral pain and is good practice in those with voiding/emptying symptoms. Positive tests should be evaluated further.
- Urodynamic investigation can provide a wide variety of information, but is not necessarily indicated for all patients.

Key references

Abrams P, Artibani W, Cardozo L et al. Reviewing the ICS 2002 terminology report: the ongoing debate. *Neurourol Urodyn* 2009;28:287.

Abrams P, Cardozo L, Fall M et al. The standardisation of terminology in lower urinary tract function: report from the standardisation sub-committee of the International Continence Society. *Urology* 2003; 61:37–49.

Goode PS, Burgio KL, Richter HE, Markland AD. Incontinence in older women. *JAMA* 2010;303:2172–81.

McLellan A, Cardozo L. Urodynamic techniques. *Int Urogynecol J Pelvic Floor Dysfunct* 2001;12:266–70.

Newman DK. Talking to patients about bladder control problems. *Nurse Pract* 2009;34:33–45.

Newman DK, Laycock J. Evaluation of the pelvic floor. In: Schussler B, Baessler FK, Moore K et al., eds. *Pelvic Floor Reeducation – Principles and Practice*, 2nd edn. London: Springer, 2008:91–104.

Rovner ES, Wein AJ. Evaluation of lower urinary tract symptoms in females. *Curr Opin Urol* 2003;13:273–8.

Sampselle CM. Teaching women to use a voiding diary. *Am J Nurs* 2003;103:62–4.

Definitions

Urinary incontinence (UI), defined as the involuntary loss of urine, is the focus of this chapter. A classification of UI is given in Table 3.1.

TABLE 3.1

Classification of urinary incontinence

Extraurethral

- Fistula (vesico-, uretero-, urethrovaginal)
- Ectopic urethra

Urethral

Functional

- Due to physical disability
- Due to lack of awareness or concern

Postvoid dribbling

- Urethral diverticulum
- Vaginal pooling of urine or blood

Outlet underactivity

- Stress urinary incontinence
  - lack of urethral support
  - urethral hypermobility
- Intrinsic sphincter deficiency
  - neurological disease/injury
  - fibrosis
- Urethral instability

Bladder overactivity

- Involuntary contractions
  - neurological disease/injury
  - bladder outlet obstruction
  - afferent activation (including inflammation/ infection)
  - idiopathic
- Decreased compliance
  - neurological disease/injury
  - fibrosis
  - idiopathic
- Combination of the above

'Overflow' incontinence

Adapted from Wein and Moy 2007.

Stress urinary incontinence (SUI) is defined as the involuntary leakage of urine on effort or exertion. Urgency incontinence is the involuntary leakage of urine accompanied, or immediately preceded, by urgency, and is largely caused by involuntary detrusor contractions (called detrusor overactivity) during bladder filling/storage. This is discussed in more detail in Chapter 4. Mixed incontinence refers to the coexistence of stress incontinence with urgency incontinence symptoms.

There are situations in which urinary incontinence cannot be considered merely as an isolated abnormality of either bladder contractility or sphincter resistance. These situations, listed in Table 3.2, are complicated to deal with because, first, they are difficult to diagnose, and, second, one entity may adversely affect or compromise treatment of the other.

Etiology

SUI suggests a problem with the bladder outlet. Urodynamic stress incontinence is noted during filling cystometry and is defined as the involuntary leakage of urine during increased abdominal pressure, in the absence of a detrusor contraction.

SUI is often divided etiologically, especially in women, into SUI due to urethral hypermobility and that due to intrinsic sphincter deficiency (ISD). Hypermobility-related SUI implies the outlet is closed at rest and opens because of the lack of a supporting scaffold underneath (backboard) against which the urethra is normally compressed during increases in intra-abdominal pressure. The lack of support and, therefore, compression is what causes the leakage and results in

---

TABLE 3.2

Combined problems associated with incontinence

- Detrusor overactivity with outlet obstruction
- Detrusor overactivity with impaired bladder contractility
- Sphincteric incontinence with impaired bladder contractility
- Sphincteric incontinence with detrusor overactivity

Adapted from Wein and Moy 2007.

urethral hypermobility. ISD implies the bladder neck and proximal urethra are not normal at rest (lack the normal closure pressure necessary to prevent exertional leakage). The bladder outlet that is damaged or diseased and fixed in an entirely open position represents the most extreme form of ISD. In reality, some ISD must exist for SUI to occur and thus sphincteric incontinence in the woman is generally due to a combination of hypermobility (lack of support) and ISD in variable proportions. Pure ISD can exist in women, and it is generally the cause of postprostatectomy sphincter incontinence in men, in whom no counterpart of hypermobility or poor support exists.

Epidemiology

The prevalence of UI in women is difficult to estimate, and differs according to the setting studied. Prevalence of UI in American community-dwelling women increases with age, from 19% at age younger than 45 years to 29% in age 80 years and older; the rate levels off from 50 to 70 years, after which prevalence again increases. Estimates vary from 5% among women aged 15 years and older in Belgium, to 69% among women aged 19 years and older in Wales. The type of incontinence also varies with age. In surveys of older women, mixed and urgency incontinence predominate, whereas stress incontinence is generally the dominant symptom in young and middle-aged women. Most women manage UI on their own, with the minority (30–45%) seeking medical help.

The prevalence of UI in men has been reported to range from 3% to 39%, with moderate/severe incontinence at 4.5%. It is generally agreed that the prevalence is less than half that in women. Urgency incontinence predominates (40–80%), followed by mixed urinary incontinence (10–30%) and stress urinary incontinence (less than 10%).

In general, the prevalence of UI in nursing-home residents is about 50% in both sexes.

Quality of life

UI has a major impact on quality of life, measured using both general and specific questionnaires (see Table 2.2, page 20). It primarily affects self-esteem, ability to maintain an independent lifestyle, social interactions with friends and family, activities of daily life, and sexual activity.

Risk factors

The risk factors identified for UI are described in the following sections.

Women

Obstetric factors can contribute to the development of UI. The effects of pregnancy and mode of delivery on urinary function are discussed in more detail in Chapter 10 (see pages 112–15).

Pregnancy. UI is common during pregnancy and usually resolves in the postpartum period. However, it has been shown to be a predictor for postpartum incontinence, as well as a risk factor for incontinence 5 years after delivery.

Delivery. There is growing evidence that vaginal delivery may predispose women to incontinence. Vaginal delivery has been shown to cause pelvic neuropathy, and other factors may include avulsion injuries to the pelvic ligaments. Studies into the mode of delivery have generally shown that, compared with nulliparous women, the risk of incontinence increases progressively, less with Cesarean section and more with vaginal delivery and forceps delivery. There is also a suggestion that higher birth weights may predispose the mother to incontinence, the risk increasing with birth weights above 4 kg.

Menopause and reproductive hormones. While it has long been considered that reduction in estrogen levels at the menopause causes atrophic changes that can lead to urinary symptoms, the literature is inconsistent in describing the role of the menopause and estrogen loss as significant contributors to UI. There is no convincing evidence for a role of hormone replacement therapy in the management of incontinence but the clinical use of vaginal estrogens (cream, tablet or ring) for symptoms of an overactive bladder is common.

Obesity is well established as a factor that contributes to the incidence of UI. It is believed that excessive weight has similar effects to pregnancy, causing chronic strain, stretching and weakening of the pelvic floor muscles and nerves. Weight loss, even a moderate amount, may decrease incontinence.

Smoking and chronic pulmonary disease are associated with chronic cough and can precipitate stress UI or worsen existing UI. There may also be an association between nicotine and increased detrusor contractions. Giving the patient information about the contribution of smoking to UI may provide a further deterrent for this unhealthy habit.

Men. Risk factors for SUI in men include age, neurological disease, urinary infection, outlet obstruction, functional and cognitive impairment, and prostatectomy.

Prostatectomy is a well-known cause of incontinence in men. The incidence of stress incontinence following transurethral resection of the prostate is about 1% and is 5–20% after radical prostatectomy.

Diagnosis and assessment

Diagnosis is largely as described in Chapter 2. A detailed clinical history is crucial in any patient with SUI in order to obtain an accurate diagnosis, and should include assessment of filling and storage symptoms as described in Chapter 2. Physical examination is also important, but neurological examination is rarely relevant, as most neurological abnormalities will be obvious when a patient first presents.

Further investigations may be necessary to elucidate the cause of SUI; the investigations carried out will to some extent depend on the facilities available and can include frequency/volume bladder records and dipstick urinalysis. Urodynamic assessment is appropriate for all patients in whom surgical treatment is being considered and in patients with complex symptoms that do not respond to simple behavioral or conservative measures or drug treatments.

Management in women

Treatment should initially be conservative and can be implemented without recourse to urodynamic assessment.

Lifestyle. Encouraging weight reduction and smoking cessation (largely to reduce cough), treating chronic cough conditions and rectifying exacerbating conditions such as constipation can all help in the management of incontinence.

Reduction in caffeine intake decreases incontinence episodes and helps with other conservative measures.

Pelvic floor muscle exercises. The pelvic floor muscles support the bladder neck, rectum and vagina (Figure 3.1). Exercises to strengthen the pelvic floor, and therefore improve support of the bladder neck, were first described by Dr Arnold Kegel in 1948. The aims are to promote patient awareness and to improve the contractility and coordination of pelvic floor muscles, especially in women with weak pelvic floor muscles.

Exercise regimens concentrate on both contraction strength and muscle endurance. The exercises described in Table 3.3 should be taught by a healthcare professional who has expertise in behavioral treatment for pelvic floor disorders (e.g. nurse specialist, physiotherapist). A pelvic floor muscle assessment should be performed to ensure correct technique. Improvement should be observed within 2–4 months.

Biofeedback training, which uses instruments to convert the effect of a pelvic floor muscle contraction into a visual or auditory response, allows patients and healthcare professionals to observe improvement in strength and bulk of the pelvic floor muscle in an objective manner. A sensor, or probe, is placed in the vagina or rectum, or skin-surface sensors are placed externally, to measure pelvic floor muscle contraction or relaxation. The measurement is presented as a numerical value that is translated into a graph (Figure 3.2). Biofeedback therapy uses either electromyography (EMG) or manometric pressure. EMG charts the electrical activity of a muscle during contraction and relaxation.

Pelvic floor muscle or transvaginal electrical stimulation with an electrode (vaginal, rectal, skin surface) can be useful if the initial pelvic floor muscle contraction is weak. This treatment is initially started in the clinic or medical office followed by a prescribed home program using a battery-operated unit. The patient can use the device for 20 minutes a day at home and adjust the strength of

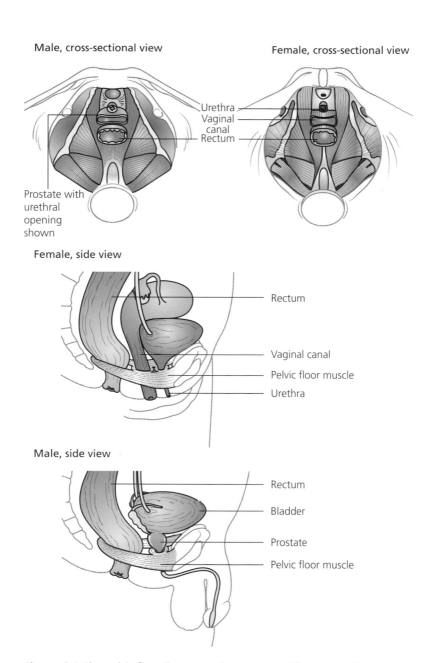

Figure 3.1 The pelvic floor (levator ani) muscle provides support for the bladder neck, vagina and rectum. Weakness in the muscle can contribute to stress incontinence.

TABLE 3.3

How to perform pelvic floor muscle exercises

- Sit in a comfortable position with your knees slightly apart
- Imagine you are in an elevator full of people and you feel the urge to pass gas so you tighten or pull in the ring of muscle around your rectum – your pelvic muscle. You should feel a lifting sensation in the area
- You should be aware of a tightening or pulling in sensation around the back passage (the rectum) and, in women, a lifting sensation in the vagina
- You should not move or tense your stomach, buttocks or thighs at all
- After tightening the muscle, relax it. You have now completed one contraction
- There are two types of pelvic floor muscle contractions – short (2 second) or quick contractions and slow (3, 5 or 10 seconds) or long contractions
  - do the short or quick muscle contractions: contract or tighten the muscle quickly and hard, and immediately relax it
  - do the slow or long (sustained) contractions: contract or tighten the muscle and hold for a count of 3, 5 or 10 seconds (as prescribed), then relax the muscle completely
- When beginning to exercise, you may only be able to do the long contractions for a few seconds
- Both types of contractions need to be repeated at least 8–10 times, giving a 5–10 second period of recovery between each repetition
- Exercises should only take around 10 minutes and should be performed at least twice a day
- Concentrate and tighten only the pelvic floor muscle. Do not tighten thighs, buttocks or stomach. If you feel your stomach move, then you are also using these muscles. Do not hold your breath. Breathe normally and/or count out loud as you exercise

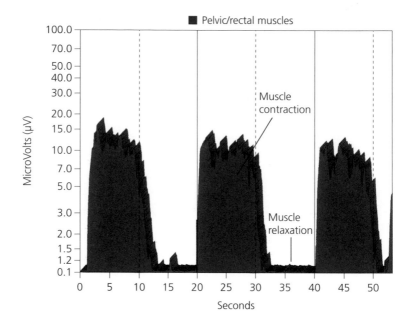

Figure 3.2 Sample biofeedback graph of pelvic floor muscle contraction and relaxation.

stimulation herself. Stimulation is delivered via vaginal or rectal sensors or skin electrodes.

Weighted vaginal cones can help women to identify the muscles of the pelvic floor (Figure 3.3). Cones of increasing weight (20–90 g) are inserted into the vagina and the woman contracts and trains her muscles to prevent the cone from falling out. Subjective improvement rates can be as high as 70%.

Pharmacological treatment

Duloxetine hydrochloride is a combined serotonin and norepinephrine (noradrenaline) reuptake inhibitor which is approved in Europe for the treatment of stress incontinence in women. Duloxetine is thought to work by increasing the tone of the urethral sphincter during filling/storage via its action on serotonin and norepinephrine in the spinal cord. Duloxetine can be used to treat moderate-to-severe stress incontinence, and has been shown to reduce

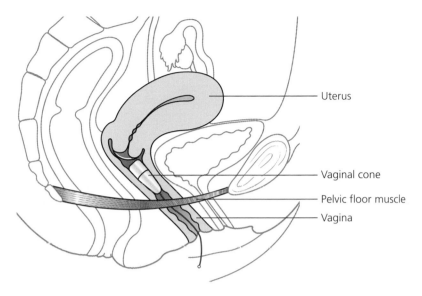

    —— Uterus

    —— Vaginal cone
    —— Pelvic floor muscle
    —— Vagina

Figure 3.3 Vaginal cones are designed to help women develop awareness of the pelvic floor muscles and to strengthen the muscles. Starting with the lightest cone, the woman has to contract the pelvic floor muscles to keep the cone in position.

the frequency of episodes of leakage. It may be more effective if combined with pelvic floor muscle exercises. Duloxetine is approved for use in Europe but not in the USA.

Surgery for stress incontinence in women should be considered only after the cause of the incontinence has been definitely ascertained. Women need to be adequately counseled about the risks and benefits of surgery for stress incontinence so that they can make an informed decision before embarking on this sort of surgery.

    Surgery for stress incontinence has changed over the last 10 years with the advent of minimally invasive techniques. The gold-standard procedure for treating stress incontinence used to be colposuspension (described below), which is major surgery that necessitates a lengthy hospital stay and has a prolonged recovery time.

    Minimally invasive mid-urethral sling insertion (Figure 3.4) is popular, as the procedure can usually be carried out on a day-case

41

(a)

(b)

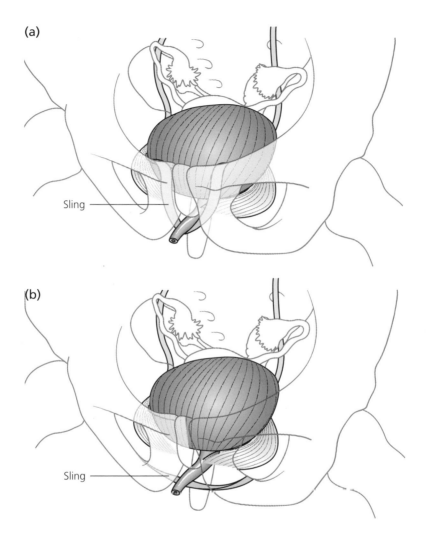

Sling

Sling

Figure 3.4 Positions of (a) retropubic and (b) transobturator mid-urethral slings to provide support for the urethra.

(outpatient) basis, complication rates are low and long-term results are excellent (up to 70–80% cure rate at up to 10 years). A number of different types of sling are available and are associated with varying degrees of success.

The principle underlying the procedure is that stress incontinence is caused by failure of the pubourethral ligaments. The sling provides support (basically a backboard) under the urethra without lifting it from its anatomic position. Tension-free vaginal tape (TVT) has been most fully evaluated, and long-term follow-up data are available. The tape is made from a monofilament polypropylene knitted mesh with a large pore size. In the original technique, the sling was placed under the mid-urethra and the ends tunneled through the retropubic space (see Figure 3.4a) without fixation, the tape being held in position by the tissues until it becomes incorporated. However, major complications such as bowel and vascular injuries have been reported, and perforation of the bladder was not uncommon (it could be managed by repositioning of the needles and postoperative bladder drainage). Other complications can include erosion of the mesh through the vagina and urethra.

A retropubic sling can also be constructed from rectus fascia or fascia lata. Success rates are the same, but overall morbidity is higher. There are a few circumstances in which autologous fascia may be preferable. Note that fascial slings are not commonly used in the UK.

The transobturator mid-urethral sling (see Figure 3.4b) was introduced to overcome some of the problems described above. The sling is placed in a similar way to the TVT but the ends of the tape are tunneled through the obturator foramen instead of going through the retropubic space. The main advantage of this technique is that the abdominal cavity is never entered, therefore decreasing the risk of bowel injury. There are few long-term follow-up data on this method as yet, and it is not known whether the reduction in the rate of bowel injury may be negated by reduced success rates and postoperative nerve pain.

Other types of sling are also available. It is worth noting that complication rates are higher with tapes made from materials other than polypropylene. For this reason, the UK's National Institute for Health and Clinical Excellence (NICE) has recommended that all slings for the treatment of stress incontinence should be composed of type 1 polypropylene mesh (knitted meshes with a large pore size).

Colposuspension provides long-term cure in 70–80% of women at 10 years. It involves elevating the bladder neck by placing sutures between the lateral vaginal fornices and the ileopectineal ligament on the back of the pubic symphysis, and can be performed via an abdominal incision or laparoscopically. One of the benefits of colposuspension is that it elevates the anterior vaginal wall and is therefore appropriate when incontinence is associated with a mild or moderate cystocele. However, it is a more invasive procedure than sling insertion, and is associated with higher rates of enterocele formation and voiding dysfunction in the postoperative period.

Most would agree that sling insertion or colposuspension should be postponed for women who want to have more children.

Injection of bulking agents (Figure 3.5) into the urethra aids continence by opposing the walls of the urethra. Agents that can be used include collagen and silicone particles suspended in a viscous gel (Macroplastique). In the past, phenol, Teflon and fat have been used, but with poor results. A number of new materials have recently been introduced or are under development.

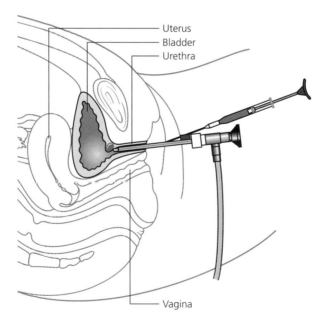

Uterus
Bladder
Urethra

Vagina

Figure 3.5 Injection of bulking agent. The agent (purple color) is injected just beneath the mucosa of the urethra at the level of the bladder neck and proximal urethra, closing the bladder neck and restoring urinary continence.

Bulking agents can be injected under local anesthesia and provide a treatment for women who are unfit to undergo general anesthesia or for whom a sling insertion or colposuspension are not suitable. Success rates are around 25–50% (lower than with mid-urethral slings and colposuspension), and the procedure may need to be repeated.

Other procedures. Historically a number of other operations have been used to treat stress incontinence in women. These include:

- anterior repair
- Stamey procedure
- Marshall–Marchetti–Krantz (MMK) procedure.

These procedures are rarely performed nowadays because the success rates and complications are worse than with minimally invasive sling insertion and colposuspension.

Complications. All surgical procedures for stress incontinence carry the risk of voiding problems in the postoperative period. Patients may be unable to pass urine or completely empty their bladders for days or weeks after surgery. A number of different methods of management are available should this occur. A temporary indwelling urethral or suprapubic catheter can be placed until the bladder recovers, or the patient can be taught intermittent self-catheterization (see Chapter 9, pages 102–4). If the patient experiences voiding difficulty after TVT insertion, it is possible to loosen the tape in the early postoperative period (within 10 days), which usually resolves the problem.

Detrusor overactivity, causing urgency, frequency and urgency incontinence, may be precipitated or worsened as a result of surgery for stress incontinence, particularly in women with bladder outlet obstruction. It is therefore important that women with mixed symptoms receive adequate counseling before consenting to surgery.

Management of stress/sphincteric incontinence in men

Stress incontinence after radical prostatectomy usually improves spontaneously. Initial management involves strengthening the pelvic floor musculature with exercises (see Table 3.3, page 39). Most patients improve over a period of weeks or months without the need for further investigation or treatment. Any patient who is still experiencing incontinence 12 months after prostatectomy should have their sphincter function investigated urodynamically. If a clinical and urodynamic diagnosis of sphincter weakness is confirmed and the bladder storage capacity is adequate at low pressure, the treatment options are:

- injection of bulking agents into the sphincter
- perineal sling
- insertion of an artificial urinary sphincter.

Injectable bulking agents can be used to treat male stress incontinence. Injection suburothelially just distal to the bladder neck by cystoscopy may close the urethra sufficiently to provide continence without affecting voiding. Reported results vary from surgeon to surgeon, but are generally less good than with the sling or sphincter, with less durability.

Perineal sling. This minimally invasive procedure involves placing a minimally compressive sling at the level of the bulbar urethra. Two absorbable tensioning sutures are threaded into the length of the mesh to fixate the mesh, allowing for flat coaptation of the urethra. Success rates with this sling in men following radical prostatectomy range from 39% to 80%, with few complications. The most common complications with perineal sling are infection and erosion.

Artificial urinary sphincter. Insertion of an artificial urinary sphincter (Figure 3.6) is a definitive treatment for intractable stress incontinence after prostatectomy, provided that the bladder pressure during filling is normal and that the patient is sufficiently fit to undergo surgery and is able to operate the artificial sphincter. Fitting of a sphincter should not be considered, except for special circumstances, for at least 1 year after prostatectomy. It is activated about 6 weeks after insertion, allowing time for the tissue around the cuff to settle and for the natural capsule around each of the components to form. When the sphincter is activated, the patient has to learn to use the sphincter by compressing the pump that causes the cuff to empty. It will then automatically refill from the reservoir over a period of 1–3 minutes.

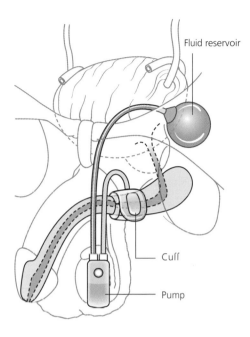

Fluid reservoir

Cuff

Pump

Figure 3.6 The artificial urinary sphincter. The sphincter cuff fits around the bladder neck or urethra and fills with fluid when activated, thereby passively compressing the urethra. To allow voiding, the pump is squeezed two or three times to open the cuff and transfer the fluid to the reservoir. The cuff automatically refills within 1–3 minutes.

The most common complications with artificial urinary sphincters are infection, erosion and mechanical problems, although these problems are becoming less common as the materials and devices improve.

Key points – urinary incontinence

- Stress incontinence is the involuntary leakage of urine on exertion. It is far more common in women than in men.
- Risk factors for stress incontinence in women include pregnancy, childbirth, menopause and obesity. Prostatectomy is the main cause in men.
- Behavioral modification, including pelvic floor muscle exercises, is effective in women and men when taught correctly, and a number of devices are available to assist with training.
- The surgical procedure of choice in women is insertion of a retropubic or transobturator tape mid-urethral sling to provide support for the urethra.
- Other alternatives in women are colposuspension and injection of bulking agents.
- Options for management in men include injection of bulking agent into the urethral sphincter, insertion of a perineal sling or artificial urinary sphincter.

Key references

Danforth KN, Townsend MK, Lifford K et al. Risk factors for urinary incontinence among middle-aged women. *Am J Obstet Gynecol* 2006;194:339–45.

Gousse AE, Madjar S, Lambert MM, Fishman IJ. Artificial urinary sphincter for post-radical prostatectomy urinary incontinence: long-term subjective results. *J Urol* 2001;166:1755–8.

Hendrix SL, Cochrane BB, Nygaard IE et al. Effects of estrogen with and without progestin on urinary incontinence. *JAMA* 2005;293:935–48.

Holroyd-Leduc JM, Tannenbaum C, Thorpe KE, Straus SE. What type of urinary incontinence does this woman have? *JAMA* 2008;299:1446–56.

Keegan PE, Atiemo K, Cody JD et al. Periurethral injection therapy for urinary incontinence in women. *Cochrane Database Syst Rev* 2007(3):CD003881.

Landefeld CS, Bowers BJ, Feld AD et al. National Institutes of Health state-of-the-science conference statement: prevention of fecal and urinary incontinence in adults. *Ann Intern Med* 2008;148:449–58.

Latthe PM, Foon R, Toozs-Hobson P. Transobturator and retropubic tape procedures in stress urinary incontinence: a systematic review and meta-analysis of effectiveness and complications. *BJOG* 2007;114:522–31.

Markland AD, Goode PS, Redden DT et al. Prevalence of urinary incontinence in men: results from the national health and nutrition examination survey. *J Urol* 2010;184:1022–7.

National Institute for Health and Clinical Excellence. Urinary incontinence: the management of urinary incontinence in women. *Clinical Guideline 40*. London: NICE, October 2006. Available from www.nice.org.uk/cg40, last accessed 25 Jan 2011.

Reynolds WS, Patel R, Msezane L et al. Current use of artificial urinary sphincters in the United States. *J Urol* 2007;178:578–83.

Richter HE, Albo ME, Zyczynski HM et al. Retropubic versus transobturator midurethral slings for stress incontinence. *N Engl J Med* 2010;362:2066–76.

Rogers RG. Clinical practice. Urinary stress incontinence in women. *N Engl J Med* 2008;358:1029–36.

Rortveit G, Daltveit AK, Hannestad YS, Hunskaar S. Urinary incontinence after vaginal delivery or cesarean section. *N Engl J Med* 2003;348:900–7.

Subak LL, Wing R, West DS et al. Weight loss to treat urinary incontinence in overweight and obese women. *N Engl J Med* 2009;360:481–90.

Wein AJ, Moy ML. Voiding function, dysfunction and urinary incontinence. In: Hanno P, Wein AJ, Malkowicz SB, eds. *Penn Clinical Manual of Urology*. Philadelphia: Saunders/Elsevier, 2007:341–478.

4 The overactive bladder and urgency incontinence

The term 'overactive bladder' (OAB) is defined as urgency, with or without urgency incontinence, usually with frequency and nocturia. The incidence of symptomatic OAB varies with age, from about 5% in those aged 18–44 years to 20% in those over 44 years of age. Although historically thought of as a condition in women, the prevalence of OAB is in fact only slightly lower in men than in women. A greater proportion of women with OAB have urgency incontinence (OAB-wet) than do men, who predominantly have OAB without incontinence (OAB-dry).

The term detrusor overactivity refers to a urodynamic observation of involuntary detrusor contractions during the filling phase, which may be spontaneous or provoked. It can only be diagnosed after urodynamic investigation. Not all patients with symptoms of OAB will be found to have detrusor overactivity, and not all patients with detrusor overactivity will have symptoms of bladder overactivity.

Etiology

Overactivity can be the result of neurological abnormalities in which involuntary detrusor contractions (detrusor overactivity) occur in the presence of underlying neuropathy (e.g. multiple sclerosis, Parkinson's disease, stroke, spinal cord injury or spina bifida).

Bladder overactivity can also be idiopathic, occurring in a neurologically normal individual. This is by far the most common category but, as the name implies, it is not fully understood. Overactivity is seen commonly in association with bladder outlet obstruction (i.e. together with prostatic obstruction in men, or after surgery for incontinence in women).

Investigation

It is important to exclude causes such as urinary tract infection (UTI), which can be detected with a urine dipstick test and culture if indicated. A frequency/volume bladder record or diary (see Figure 2.3, page 21) is a reliable method of quantifying urinary frequency and volume. It also gives a good indication of fluid intake. Diaries should be kept for at least 3 days to allow for variations in normal activities, but the ideal duration is not known. The diary for a patient with OAB will show frequent, irregular, small-volume voids.

Urodynamic studies are rarely indicated initially in patients who have symptoms suggestive of OAB, and most patients receive empirical treatment (drugs and or behavioral) whether or not urodynamic studies show detrusor overactivity. The only real role for these tests in patients with OAB symptoms is if conservative therapy fails and more invasive treatment is contemplated.

Urodynamic investigation is necessary for the diagnosis of detrusor overactivity. The classic findings on multichannel cystometry are involuntary increases in detrusor pressure during filling. It is important to note, however, that only approximately 50% of patients with symptoms of detrusor overactivity will have an abnormality on supine slow-filling cystometry. If symptoms suggest detrusor overactivity but filling cystometry reveals a stable bladder, additional provocative procedures during filling, such as coughing and changes in posture, may reveal detrusor overactivity. A typical cystometry trace from a patient with detrusor overactivity is shown in Figure 2.5, page 28.

Management

Behavioral therapy (sometimes referred to as 'conservative treatment') helps an individual change habits to modify bladder symptoms and learn training techniques to control symptoms of bladder dysfunction. They include lifestyle changes or so-called 'self-care practices' and bladder training, urgency suppression and pelvic floor muscle training exercises.

Lifestyle changes
Alteration in fluid intake. There is a common misconception that a fluid intake of up to 3 liters/day is needed for good health, and this becomes apparent in the frequency/volume bladder records of many

patients. Reduction in fluid intake can bring about a dramatic improvement in patients with OAB. However, many patients with OAB will report too severe a restriction of daily fluid intake which is also not a good practice. The ideal fluid intake for an adult is approximately 1500 mL or 30 mL/kg bodyweight per 24 hours.

Reduction in caffeine intake. A trial of caffeine-intake reduction is indicated in all patients presenting with OAB symptoms. It is worth noting that caffeine is present in tea, cola and chocolate, as well as coffee. See Table 4.1 for specific foods and beverages that patients should consider reducing to determine the effect on OAB symptoms.

Weight loss. There is evidence to suggest that weight loss, even a moderate amount of 5 to 10%, can help with the symptoms of OAB in overweight patients. It is therefore worth advising weight loss to any patient who has a body mass index above 30 kg/m².

TABLE 4.1

Dietary modifications* that may help overactive bladder

- Alcoholic beverages
- Milk/milk products
- Carbonated beverages
- Caffeinated products such as coffee, tea, soft drinks (only drink 'caffeine-free'), energy drinks, chocolate†
- Citrus juices and fruits
- Highly spiced foods, tomato-based products
- Sugar, honey
- Corn syrup
- Artificial sweetener (aspartame)

*A significant rise in detrusor pressure with bladder filling has been demonstrated with caffeine so eliminating foods and liquids containing caffeine can decrease symptoms of an overactive bladder. The effect of other foods and beverages on the bladder is not understood but elimination of one or all of the items listed may improve bladder control.
†Taper caffeine intake slowly to avoid migraine-type headache.

TABLE 4.2

High-fiber mixture to help relieve constipation

A successful way to adequately increase fiber is by using a 'special bran recipe'

- Mix together:
  - 1 cup of apple sauce
  - 1 cup of coarse unprocessed wheat bran
  - ¾ cup of prune juice
- Refrigerate mixture and take 2 tablespoons of the mixture every day
- Take the mixture in the evening for a morning bowel movement
- Increase the bran mixture by two tablespoons each week until bowel movements are regular
- Always drink one large glass of water with the mixture

Bowel regularity. Constipation and difficulty with defecation (straining during bowel movements) can cause increased pressure on the bladder, sometimes leading or contributing to overactive bladder. Individuals should avoid constipation through increased fiber, exercise and fluid. Table 4.2 provides a high fiber mixture that can be recommended for patients with constipation.

Scheduled or timed voiding means a person voids on a rigid fixed schedule (e.g. every 2–3 hours). Toileting takes place whether or not urge sensation is present and the goal is for the person to avoid urgency and incontinence.

Bladder training with urgency suppression. Individuals with OAB symptoms usually void more frequently than normal (called 'defensive voiding') because of urgency, or to avoid situations where urgency is likely to cause a problem. A toileting program, such as bladder training, can help this frequency as it uses a progressive voiding schedule combined with techniques to control and suppress urgency. In bladder training, the individual actively attempts to increase the interval between the first desire to void and the actual void. Patients are instructed to use techniques that control or suppress urgency.

Slow, deep breathing exercises relax the bladder, decrease the intensity of the urgency and delay voiding, while distraction methods involve patients in tasks that require mental concentration. The voiding interval should be increased by 15 to 30 minutes each week until an interval of at least 3 to 4 hours is achieved. Bladder training has been shown to be beneficial, and a course lasting for a minimum of 6 weeks, together with pelvic floor muscle training with exercises (see exercises in Table 3.3, page 39), should be offered as first-line treatment.

Pelvic floor muscle training. Individuals with OAB can use rapid repeated pelvic floor muscle contractions ('quick flicks') to suppress urgency and control incontinence and restore a normal voiding interval. Patients are taught to resist rushing to the bathroom when experiencing the need to void as this increases pressure in the abdomen and may actually cause a detrusor contraction. Instead, they are instructed to stay still, be seated if possible and rapidly contract their pelvic floor muscle 3 to 5 times consecutively to achieve detrusor relaxation.

Complementary therapies are treatments that are not part of the traditional OAB treatments and include acupuncture, relaxation, meditation and herbal remedies. Acupuncture has been reported to reduce symptoms in both men and women with OAB, but there is a lack of controlled studies and skilled practitioners.

Pharmacological therapy

Antimuscarinic drugs are the mainstay of treatment for symptoms of OAB and detrusor overactivity (Table 4.3). These drugs were thought to act by blocking the muscarinic receptors on the detrusor muscle that are stimulated by acetylcholine released by activated parasympathetic nerves, thereby reducing the ability of the bladder to contract. It should be noted, however, that these drugs work mainly during the storage phase, decreasing urgency and increasing bladder capacity, when there is normally no parasympathetic input into the lower urinary tract. All these agents have been shown to decrease afferent (sensory) neural traffic during filling/storage. Current thinking is that these agents act primarily on the sensory side at lower dosages. As the dosage increases, actions on the motor side may become apparent.

TABLE 4.3

Antimuscarinic agents used in the treatment of overactive bladder

Drug	Chemical structure and primary action	Usual dosage
Darifenacin	Tertiary amine	7.5 or 15 mg once daily
Fesoterodine	Tertiary amine	4 or 8 mg once daily
Oxybutynin	Tertiary amine Some calcium antagonist properties	Immediate release: 2.5 or 5 mg twice or three times daily Sustained release: 5–30 mg once daily (titratable) Transdermal patch: replace twice weekly, provides 3.9 mg per day Transdermal gel: 1 g unit dose applied once daily delivers ~4 mg oxybutynin
Propiverine*	Tertiary amine Balanced muscarinic receptor antagonist Some calcium antagonist properties	15 mg twice or three times daily
Solifenacin	Tertiary amine	5 or 10 mg once daily
Tolterodine	Tertiary amine	Immediate release: 1 or 2 mg twice daily Sustained release: 4 mg once daily
Trospium	Quaternary amine	Immediate release: 20 mg twice daily Sustained release: 60 mg once daily

*Not licensed in the USA.

The effects of antimuscarinic drugs in patients with OAB symptoms are shown in Table 4.4. Treatment should be for 2–4 weeks in the first

TABLE 4.4

Effects of antimuscarinic drugs in patients with overactive bladder symptoms

- Decrease in episodes of urgency and urgency incontinence
- Increase in bladder volume before the first involuntary bladder contraction
- Decrease in urgency frequency
- Increase in total bladder capacity
- Improved quality of life

instance and can be continued if there is benefit and the side effects are tolerable; however, there is lack of evidence for how long treatment should be continued. Research has shown that combining drug therapy with behavioral treatment will produce the best outcome in terms of reduction in OAB symptoms. Many recommend discontinuing the drug after some months to determine whether bladder training has occurred and symptoms are improved.

The side effects of antimuscarinic drugs may include dry mouth, constipation and nausea, and are generally mild to moderate. Less commonly, blurred vision, cognitive dysfunction and changes in mental state may occur. The elderly, especially the frail elderly, should be followed with this last possibility in mind. Antimuscarinics are contraindicated in patients with closed angle glaucoma or myasthenia gravis. Caution is advised in patients with significant bladder outlet obstruction and pre-existing constipation.

Patients should be counseled on how to deal with side effects and given written information about the drug and simple management strategies. Suggestions to counter a dry mouth include chewing sugar-free gum, sucking on sugar-free hard candy and using saliva-producing dental products. Healthcare professionals should recommend strategies for avoiding constipation, including adequate fluid intake, adequate dietary fiber or psyllium-based fiber supplements, regular exercise, avoidance of laxatives and advice for regular bowel habits.

Oxybutynin is the most commonly used antimuscarinic. Initially it was available as an immediate-release preparation, at a dose of 2.5–5 mg three times daily. Extended-release oxybutynin delivers the drug at a constant rate over a 24-hour period and can be given in doses of 5–30 mg daily. It has a better side-effect profile than the immediate-release formulation.

Transdermal administration of oxybutynin avoids first-pass liver metabolism and improves tolerability. Patches deliver a dose of 3.9 mg daily and are replaced twice weekly. Topical gel is used daily.

Second-generation oral antimuscarinics (e.g. darifenacin, fesoterodine, solifenacin and tolterodine) were developed to reduce the side effects experienced with oral oxybutynin while maintaining their clinical effectiveness. These drugs are taken once daily, which helps with compliance. All of these, except tolterodine, have two dosages, which allows for dose titration to increase effectiveness.

Treatment with a second-generation antimuscarinic should, ideally, last for at least 4 to 6 weeks to determine effectiveness. For the titratable (two dosage) agents, opinion is divided as to when a decision should be made regarding uptitration (2 to 4 weeks). Effectiveness seems roughly similar between products, producing 60–75% reduction in urgency incontinence episodes. If no benefit is seen, urodynamic studies should be performed before contemplating more invasive treatments.

Botulinum toxin (BTX) has the potential to revolutionize the management of refractory detrusor overactivity. It is injected directly into the detrusor muscle or suburothelially via a cystoscope (Figure 4.1), under local or general anesthesia, and acts by inhibiting neurotransmitter release, which decreases muscle contractility. There are two subtypes of BTX: BTX-A and BTX-B; the former is more widely used. BTX has been shown to be effective in the treatment of detrusor overactivity within 1–2 weeks of administration. The effect is reversible, and regeneration takes place over a period of 5–9 months, which means that repeated injections may be necessary. The most important potential adverse effects are detrusor hypotonia and urinary retention. Although widely used, BTX does not yet have regulatory approval for this indication in the USA or the UK, but trials

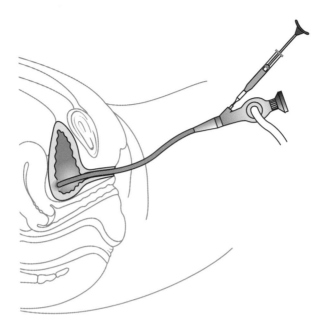

Figure 4.1 Botulinum toxin is injected via a cystoscope directly into the detrusor muscle.

are in progress. The exact dosage, number of injections per treatment and sites of injection for neurogenic and idiopathic OAB have yet to be standardized.

Neuromodulation involves the electrical stimulation of a peripheral nerve or the sacral spinal nerve roots and is thought to improve the ability to suppress detrusor contractions. It is being used increasingly in the treatment of refractory detrusor overactivity. The various techniques for neuromodulation include removable peripheral nerve stimulators and implantable sacral nerve stimulators performed in two stages. Overall, electrical neurostimulation and neuromodulation have a 30–50% clinical success rate.

Sacral nerve stimulation (Figure 4.2) differs from other forms of neuromodulation in that it provides continuous stimulation via an implanted pulse generator connected to an electrode within the S3 and S4 foramina. Its mode of action is not entirely clear, but results in this

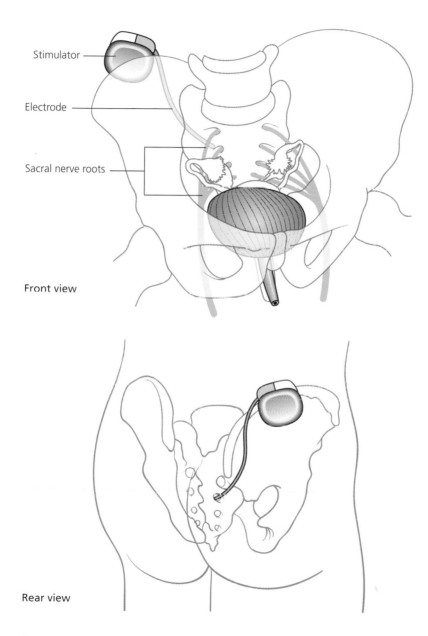

Stimulator

Electrode

Sacral nerve roots

Front view

Rear view

Figure 4.2 Sacral nerve stimulation provides continuous stimulation via an implanted pulse generator connected to an electrode within the S3 and S4 foramina.

difficult-to-treat group of patients appear promising. Sacral nerve stimulation has been shown to be safe, effective and durable. This treatment is approved for use in both Europe and the USA.

Surgery

Augmentation cystoplasty used to be the gold standard in the surgical treatment of refractory detrusor overactivity but is now rarely necessary, except in cases of neuropathic overactivity refractory to all other treatment modalities. The procedure involves opening the bladder and stitching in a piece of compliant tissue, usually a loop of detubularized ileum on a vascular pedicle, to increase the bladder capacity and compliance. The bladder remains overactive, but when it contracts the improved compliance means that lower intravesical pressures are generated, protecting the upper tracts from the effects of high intravesical pressure. Urgency incontinence is also reduced.

Because the bladder contractility is reduced, there is a high risk of postoperative urinary retention, and patients should be counseled about the possibility of self-catheterization before undergoing surgery (see pages 102–4).

When bowel has been used to augment the bladder, the mucosa continues to secrete mucus, which is passed with the urine and can lead to retention. There is also a risk of stone formation and malignant change in the transposed segment of bowel.

This procedure is most commonly used when the upper urinary tract is at risk from damage due to increased intravesical pressure, which is most common in the neuropathic bladder (see Chapter 9).

Detrusor myomectomy has recently been suggested as an alternative to augmentation cystoplasty. It involves removal of the detrusor muscle from the dome of the bladder, leaving the mucosa intact, in effect creating a large bladder diverticulum. This allows bladder capacity to increase and lowers the intravesical pressure. This technique circumvents the potential complications of mucus retention, stone formation and malignant change seen with cystoplasty. However, it is a relatively new procedure and opinion is divided as to its long-term results.

Key points – the overactive bladder and urgency incontinence

- Overactive bladder (OAB) describes a condition in which the patient experiences urgency, with or without urge incontinence, usually with frequency and nocturia.
- Detrusor overactivity refers to involuntary detrusor contractions during filling; diagnosis is by urodynamic investigation.
- Bladder overactivity can be neurogenic or idiopathic. Idiopathic OAB can be associated with bladder outlet obstruction.
- A frequency/volume bladder record is useful in diagnosis.
- Initial management includes behavioral modification.
- Antimuscarinic drugs are a mainstay of conservative treatment.
- Other options for refractory OAB are neuromodulation and augmentation cystoplasty. Intradetrusor botulinum toxin injection is under investigation and seems promising for refractory cases.

Key references

Alhasso A, Glazener CM, Pickard R, N'Dow J. Adrenergic drugs for urinary incontinence in adults. *Cochrane Database Syst Rev* 2005(3):CD001842.

Brazzelli M, Murray A, Fraser C. Efficacy and safety of sacral nerve stimulation for urinary urge incontinence: a systematic review. *J Urol* 2006;175:835–41.

Ellsworth P, Kirshenbaum E. Update on the pharmacologic management of overactive bladder: the present and the future. *Urol Nurs* 2010; 30:29–38.

MacDiarmid S, Rogers A. Male overactive bladder: the role of urodynamics and anticholinergics. *Curr Urol Rep* 2007;8:66–73.

Newman DK, Wein AJ. *Managing and Treating Urinary Incontinence*, 2nd edn. Baltimore: Health Professions Press, 2009:245–306.

Ouslander JG. Management of overactive bladder. *N Engl J Med* 2004;350:786–99.

Rosenberg MT, Newman DK, Tallman CT, Page SA. Overactive bladder: recognition requires vigilance for symptoms. *Cleve Clin J Med* 2007;74 Suppl 3:S21–9.

Schurch B. Botulinum toxin for the management of bladder dysfunction. *Drugs* 2006;66:1301–18.

Wyman JF, Burgio KL, Newman DK. Practical aspects of lifestyle modifications and behavioural interventions in the treatment of overactive bladder and urgency urinary incontinence. *Int J Clin Pract* 2009;63:1177–91.

Voiding (emptying) problems occur when there is an impediment to the normal smooth emptying of the bladder. This may result from obstruction to the normal bladder outflow – the focus of this chapter – alone or in combination with impaired contractility of the detrusor muscle. Bladder outlet obstruction may occur at any point along the length of the urethra from the bladder neck to the urethral meatus.

Etiology and risk factors

The likely causes of bladder outlet obstruction are listed in Table 5.1. The most common cause in men is benign prostatic enlargement (BPE) secondary to hyperplasia and in women, pelvic organ prolapse (POP),

TABLE 5.1

Causes of bladder outlet obstruction

Congenital
- Posterior urethral valves
- Urethral stricture
- Ectopic ureterocele

Acquired
- Structural
  - Benign prostatic enlargement
  - Prostatic carcinoma
  - Bladder neck obstruction
  - Urethral stricture
  - Urethral or bladder stones
  - External compression
  - Pelvic organ prolapse
- Functional
  - Detrusor–sphincter dyssynergia
  - Detrusor atony (contributing factor)

with kinking of the urethra. The patient may present with a variety of storage and voiding symptoms.

Benign prostatic hyperplasia (BPH) refers to a regional nodular growth of varying combinations of glandular and stromal proliferation that occurs in almost all men who have testes and who live long enough (see *Fast Facts: Benign Prostatic Hyperplasia)*. The term encompasses histological cellular proliferation (microscopic BPH) and consequent prostate enlargement (macroscopic BPH). The term BPE indicates benign prostatic enlargement, usually due to BPH, while BPO indicates benign prostatic obstruction, a common cause of bladder outlet obstruction.

Microscopic BPH is seen in about 25% of men aged 40–50 years, 50% of men aged 50–60 years, 65% of men aged 60–70 years, 80% of men aged 70–80 years and 90% of men aged 80–90 years. It is estimated that 25–50% of men with microscopic and macroscopic BPH (BPE) will develop lower urinary tract symptoms due to BPO. However, far fewer men complain about these symptoms than of BPH, and even fewer seek help because of these symptoms.

The cause of BPH is not fully understood. The hormonal theory postulates that estrogen–androgen synergism associated with aging drives prostatic growth.

Posterior urethral valves are a congenital cause of bladder outlet obstruction in boys, which, if severe, can lead to hydronephrosis and renal failure. One in every 5000–8000 boys is born with posterior urethral valves.

Urethral stricture is an abnormal narrowing of the urethra that causes obstruction to the outflow of urine and may ultimately lead to back pressure on the bladder, ureters and kidneys. Strictures may be caused by inflammation or scarring as a result of surgery, disease or injury. The risk is increased in patients with sexually transmitted diseases, repeated episodes of urethritis or BPH. Instrumentation of the urethra (with a catheter or cystoscope) also increases the risk. Congenital strictures and true strictures occur rarely in women.

Primary bladder neck obstruction is thought to occur as a result of congenital constriction, or failure to open that is not associated with the urethra. It is characterized by incomplete opening of the bladder neck during voluntary or involuntary voiding. It is found almost exclusively in young and middle-aged men, and is characterized by long-standing storage and voiding symptoms. These men typically have normal-sized prostate glands, and objective evidence of obstruction is easily obtained on urodynamic examination. Once obstruction is diagnosed, it may be located to the bladder neck by videourodynamic investigation. The diagnosis may also be made on the grounds of outlet obstruction in the absence of urethral stricture, prostatic enlargement or detrusor–sphincter dyssynergia (DSD).

Secondary bladder neck obstruction may be caused by posterior urethral valves, and results from hypertrophy of the bladder neck muscle in response to increased voiding pressure caused by the urethral abnormality.

Symptoms

Symptoms of bladder outlet obstruction vary. The most common symptoms associated with bladder outlet obstruction are listed in Table 5.2.

TABLE 5.2

Common symptoms that may be associated with bladder outlet obstruction

- Slow urinary flow
- Delayed onset of urination (urinary hesitancy)
- Inability to urinate (acute urinary retention)
- Urine stream that starts and stops (intermittent stream or intermittency)

- Urgency/frequency
- Urgency incontinence
- Nocturia
- Continuous feeling of a full bladder
- Straining to void

Examination and investigations

A thorough abdominal and pelvic examination should be carried out to evaluate the following:

- bladder distension
- abdominal mass
- prostatic enlargement and presence/absence of nodularity or induration (digital rectal examination [Figure 5.1] is mandatory in men and has been shown to be a fairly accurate predictor of prostate size but not of the presence of obstruction)
- POP, particularly cystocele, and vaginal vault in women.

In addition, urinalysis should be performed to detect hematuria (see Chapter 6) and signs of infection, and serum creatinine should be measured. Some men with BPH will have some degree of renal impairment. It is important to investigate this, as it affects clinical management. For example, a man with BPH and renal impairment may require more urgent surgical intervention and will need to be monitored more closely during and after surgery.

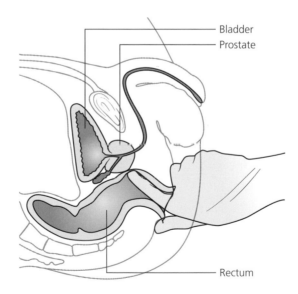

Figure 5.1 Digital rectal examination of the prostate is mandatory for men with lower urinary tract symptoms, and has been shown to be an accurate predictor of prostate size.

There is some debate about whether the measurement of prostate-specific antigen (PSA) should be mandatory. This issue is beyond the scope of this book; however, it would seem sensible to consider measuring the serum PSA in all men with a life expectancy of more than 5 years and in whom the diagnosis of prostate cancer would influence treatment decisions. Ideally, the advantages and disadvantages of such testing should be explained to the patient.

Uroflowmetry and urodynamic investigation. Measurement of urinary flow rate is an extremely useful investigation in patients with voiding dysfunction. The reduced flow rate characteristic of prostatic outlet obstruction is shown in Figure 2.4, page 26. Urodynamically, outlet obstruction is generally defined as high detrusor pressure accompanied by low urine flow rate. Once obstruction has been diagnosed, videourodynamic investigation can be useful to determine the site of the obstruction.

Urodynamic studies are not indicated for all men suspected of having BPH. They are most useful to differentiate outlet obstruction from impaired detrusor contractility, and should be performed in patients with equivocal findings in whom invasive therapy is being considered. Videourodynamic studies, with reduction of the POP, are helpful in women.

Transrectal ultrasonography can be helpful if an accurate prostate size estimate is desired and when clinical findings or PSA levels suggest the presence of prostate cancer. It is also used to guide prostatic biopsy.

Measurement of postvoid residual volume is a useful aid in the management of patients with outlet obstruction, but the amount may vary quite a lot in a given individual.

Management
Bladder outlet obstruction secondary to benign prostatic obstruction. The aim of treatment is to relieve the obstruction by reducing the smooth muscle tone or bulk of the prostate. Initial therapy for bothersome symptoms includes medications (Table 5.3).

Relatively selective α-1 adrenoceptor antagonists ('alpha blockers') have been shown to increase peak urinary flow rates and improve symptoms in 30–45% of men, but they are of little value in patients with complete inability to void. They act by relaxing the prostate and bladder neck smooth muscle, reducing outlet obstruction without adversely affecting detrusor contractility. Side effects include ejaculation issues, floppy iris syndrome, dizziness, rhinitis, headache and postural hypotension.

5α-reductase inhibitors block the conversion of testosterone to dihydrotestosterone, which plays a key role in the development of BPH. These drugs can potentially reverse or arrest the process of BPE and have been shown to reduce prostate volume by up to 20% over

TABLE 5.3

Agents used in the treatment of BPH

Drug	Chemical structure and primary action	Usual dosage
Dutasteride	5α-reductase inhibitor	0.5 mg once daily
Finasteride	5α-reductase inhibitor	5 mg once daily
Alfuzosin	α-adrenoceptor antagonist	10 mg once daily
Doxazosin	α-adrenoceptor antagonist	1–8 mg once daily
Prazosin	α-adrenoceptor antagonist	2 mg twice a day
Silodosin (not licensed in UK)	α-adrenoceptor antagonist	4 mg or 8 mg once daily with food
Tamsulosin	α-adrenoceptor antagonist	0.4 mg once daily
Terazosin	α-adrenoceptor antagonist	5 mg or 10 mg once daily

6–10 months. Side effects include erectile dysfunction, libido loss and ejaculatory disturbances.

Because they have different mechanisms of action, there is a rationale to combining alpha-blocker therapy with 5α-reductase inhibition in larger prostates (5α-reductase inhibitors are generally not used for treatment if the prostate is smaller than 30 mL).

Surgical treatment of BPH has the best results in terms of improvement in symptoms and urine flow rates, but is associated with a much higher incidence of complications than medical treatment.

Transurethral resection of the prostate (Figure 5.2) is the most common surgical treatment for BPH. The prostate is resected with a diathermy loop in a resectoscope inserted via the urethra. Symptom relief is achieved in 70–90% of men. The most significant complications are erectile dysfunction in 2–5%, incontinence in 0.2–1% and retrograde ejaculation in 70–90% of men.

Transurethral incision of the bladder neck and prostate is used when a patient has obstruction caused by a prostate that is relatively small (generally less than 35 g), with a high bladder neck and no hyperplasia of the middle lobe. The procedure involves making an incision through the bladder neck from just below the level of the

(a) (b)

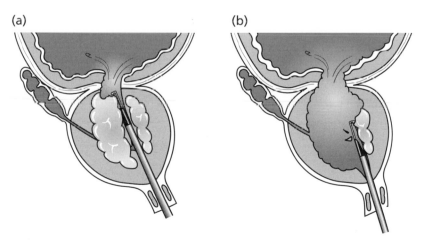

Figure 5.2 Transurethral resection of the prostate. (a) The median lobe is resected; (b) lateral adenoma tissue is removed, leaving a cavity that subsequently epithelializes over 4–6 weeks.

ureteric orifices to a point about 0.1 cm proximal to the verumontanum. It is almost as effective as transurethral resection but with lower complication rates, although the likelihood that further treatment may become necessary is higher.

Laser ablation of the prostate is an alternative to transurethral resection. It involves vaporization of the enlarged prostate with a neodynium, yttrium or holmium laser. This procedure may have advantages over the traditional transurethral resection as it causes less bleeding and the hospital stay is generally shorter, while the short-term outcomes are similar.

Open prostatectomy is indicated only in men who have extremely large prostates.

Primary bladder neck obstruction. Although α-1 adrenoceptor antagonists provide some relief in patients with bladder neck dysfunction, definitive relief is best achieved in men by bladder neck incision. Surgery should be carried out with caution in the rare woman with primary bladder neck obstruction, as the risk of postoperative urinary incontinence after bladder neck incision is high.

Urethral stricture Treatment is initially by urethral dilatation or urethrotomy, although complex or recurrent cases may require urethroplasty.

Key points – voiding problems

- Voiding problems occur when normal smooth emptying of the bladder is impeded, through obstruction or impaired detrusor contractility.
- Benign prostatic enlargement secondary to benign prostatic hyperplasia (BPH), a process of normal aging in men, is the most common cause of outlet obstruction. In women, pelvic organ prolapse (POP) can cause obstruction. Rarer causes include posterior urethral valves, urethral stricture and bladder neck obstruction, which may be congenital or secondary to increased voiding pressures as a result of urethral abnormality.
- Uroflowmetry and urodynamic investigations are useful in the diagnosis of outlet obstruction but are not indicated for all men thought to have BPH. Transurethral ultrasonography and measurement of postvoid residual volume may also provide useful information. Videourodynamic investigations can be helpful in women with POP and suspected obstruction.
- Obstruction due to BPH can be treated with α-1 adrenoceptor antagonists and 5α-reductase inhibitors. Surgery (transurethral resection, vaporization or incision of the prostate) may be needed.
- Surgery is often required for bladder neck obstruction and urethral stricture.

Key references

Barry MJ, Roehrborn CG. Benign prostatic hyperplasia. *BMJ* 2001;323:1042–6.

Fried NM. New laser treatment approaches for benign prostatic hyperplasia. *Curr Urol Rep* 2007;8:47–52.

Kirby RS, Gilling PJ. *Fast Facts: Benign Prostatic Hyperplasia*, 7th edn. Oxford: Health Press, 2011.

Madersbacher S, Marszalek M, Lackner J et al. The long-term outcome of medical therapy for BPH. *Eur Urol* 2007;51:1522–33.

McCrery RJ, Appell RA. Bladder outlet obstruction in women: iatrogenic, anatomic, and neurogenic. *Curr Urol Rep* 2006;7:363–9.

Rosenberg MT, Staskin DR, Kaplan SA et al. A practical guide to the evaluation and treatment of male lower urinary tract symptoms in the primary care setting. *Int J Clin Pract* 2007;61:1535–46.

Wein AJ, Lee DI. Benign prostatic hyperplasia and related entities. In: Hanno P, Wein AJ, Malkowicz SB, eds. *Penn Clinical Manual of Urology.* Philadelphia: Saunders/ Elsevier, 2007:479–522.

Hematuria can originate from anywhere along the urinary tract and may be an indicator of underlying pathology. It can be microscopic or macroscopic (gross), but the investigation for each is similar.

The prevalence of hematuria on urine dipstick testing in adults is estimated by various sources to be 2–16%. Dipstick testing is sensitive but is not specific, and it is sometimes difficult to distinguish between 'physiological' amounts of blood in the urine and blood that is the result of pathology.

Etiology

Urinary tract pathology is found in 2–10% of patients under the age of 50 years with microscopic hematuria. The most common pathologies are stones, infection, nephritis and, in men, prostate enlargement (see page 64). Urinary tract malignancy is rarely seen in patients under 40 years of age. Over 50 years, 10–20% of patients with microscopic hematuria will have significant urinary tract pathology. Malignancy is more common in this age group when there is gross hematuria.

History

In taking a history it is important to distinguish hematuria from rectal bleeding, and from vaginal bleeding in women. A history of urinary frequency and dysuria would suggest an infectious cause, which is the most common cause of hematuria in young women. Urinary tract calculi may present with pain. Glomerulonephritis or nephropathy may occur secondary to a recent upper respiratory tract infection, rash or edema.

Drugs may cause hematuria: non-steroidal anti-inflammatory drugs can cause papillary necrosis, while danazol and cyclophosphamide can cause hemorrhagic cystitis. Anticoagulants will not cause hematuria unless the person is over-anticoagulated.

Bladder tumors classically present with painless frank hematuria. Risk factors for bladder tumors are shown in Table 6.1.

TABLE 6.1

Risk factors for bladder tumors

- Smoking
- Exposure to chemicals or dyes (benzenes or aromatic amines)
- Chemotherapy with cyclosphosphamide or ifosfamide
- *Shistosoma haematobium* infection
- Chronic irritation and infection
- Pelvic irradiation
- Age over 40 years

Investigations

Flow charts for the investigation of hematuria , as recommended in 2001 by the American Urologic Association Best Practice Policy Panel on Asymptomatic Microhematuria in Adults are shown in Figures 6.1 and 6.2.

Microscopy. Hematuria identified by dipstick urinalysis should always be investigated further by urine microscopy. Microscopic hematuria is present if more than three red blood cells per high-power field are visible in urinary sediment from two out of three freshly voided, clean-catch midstream urine samples. The incidence of hematuria on microscopy varies from 0.2% to 16.1% in population-based studies.

Microscopy can also provide further information about the morphology of the red blood cells. Misshapen red blood cells are usually glomerular in origin, whereas normal red blood cells generally come from the lower urinary tract. Red blood cell casts are almost always associated with glomerular disease.

Urine culture is vital to exclude infection as a cause of hematuria; hematuria should never be attributed to infection without a positive culture. In the case of urine infection, a specimen should be examined after treatment to exclude continuing hematuria.

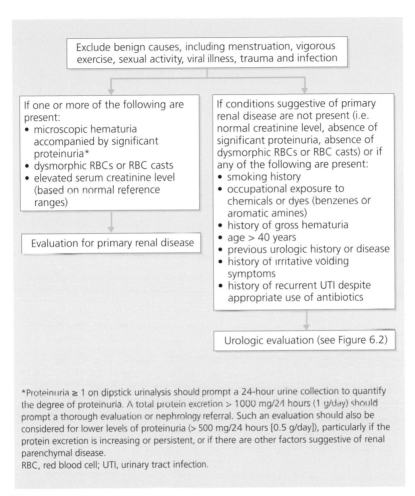

*Proteinuria ≥ 1 on dipstick urinalysis should prompt a 24-hour urine collection to quantify the degree of proteinuria. A total protein excretion > 1000 mg/24 hours (1 g/day) should prompt a thorough evaluation or nephrology referral. Such an evaluation should also be considered for lower levels of proteinuria (> 500 mg/24 hours [0.5 g/day]), particularly if the protein excretion is increasing or persistent, or if there are other factors suggestive of renal parenchymal disease.
RBC, red blood cell; UTI, urinary tract infection.

Figure 6.1 Initial evaluation of patients with newly diagnosed asymptomatic microscopic hematuria. The recommended definition of microscopic hematuria is three or more red blood cells per high-power field on microscopic evaluation of two of three properly collected specimens. Adapted from Grossfeld et al. 2001.

Biochemistry. Urine should be tested for proteinuria, which may be a sign of renal pathology or an extrarenal medical disorder. If proteinuria is identified, serum urea, creatinine and electrolytes should be measured.

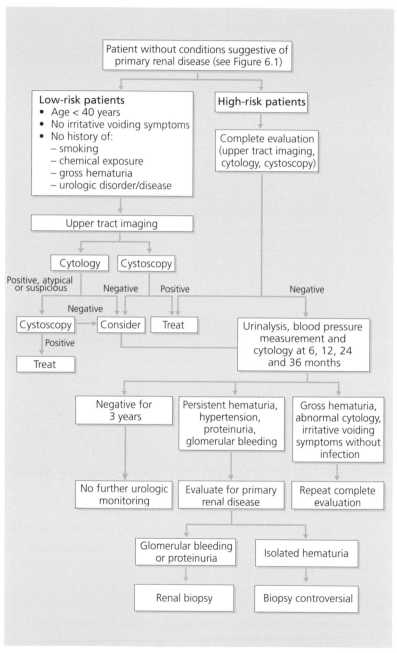

Figure 6.2 Diagnosis of hematuria in patients without conditions suggestive of primary renal disease. Adapted from Grossfeld et al. 2001.

Urine cytology is helpful in the diagnosis of transitional cell carcinoma. It is important to note, however, that sensitivity varies from less than 20% to over 90% depending on the tumor grade, sensitivity being lowest for well-differentiated tumors.

Imaging

Ultrasonography of the renal tract is the preferred initial imaging technique for identifying renal parenchymal disease, hydronephrosis and stone fragments. If hydronephrosis is found, the entire renal tract should be investigated. Ultrasonography can be used to detect and characterize renal masses but is unreliable in detecting upper tract urothelial tumors.

Plain abdominal radiography is useful to detect calcification due to renal tract stones, which affect about 5% of the population. Calcification may also be seen with infection such as tuberculosis, and nephrocalcinosis.

Intravenous urography (IVU) was traditionally the modality of choice for imaging the urinary tract, and some still consider it to be the best imaging test for the initial evaluation of microscopic hematuria. It has limited sensitivity for the detection of small renal masses and cannot differentiate between solid and cystic masses.

CT is more sensitive for detecting small renal masses, and is the investigation of choice for detecting renal tract stones – it is extremely sensitive (94–98%) compared with IVU (52–59%) and ultrasonography (19%). CT is used to detect and characterize solid renal masses as well as renal and perirenal infections and associated complications. CT is therefore the most efficient investigation in differentiating the causes of hematuria and, if used as the investigation of first choice, would reduce the time taken to diagnose the underlying etiology. The sensitivity of CT with urographic follow through (CT urography) in detecting urothelial lesions compared with IVU is not yet established.

Cystoscopy is recommended for the investigation of hematuria in adults. It allows for accurate detection of mucosal abnormalities and can be performed reliably with a flexible or rigid cystoscope under local anesthesia. It is possible to take bladder biopsies using a flexible cystoscope, although resection requires a rigid cystoscope and general anesthesia.

'One-stop' clinics. In European countries, the investigation of hematuria is often carried out in 'one-stop' clinics with facilities for cytology, ultrasonography and flexible cystoscopy, the aim being to make the diagnosis in a single outpatient visit.

Management

The main principles of managing hematuria are as follows.
- Infections should be managed appropriately.
- Patients with stones or renal tumors should be referred to the appropriate urologist.
- Patients with significant proteinuria, renal insufficiency, or red blood cell casts or dysmorphic red blood cells on microscopy should be referred to a nephrologist for evaluation of renal parenchymal disease, which may necessitate a percutaneous renal biopsy.

Follow-up. Investigation finds no cause for microscopic hematuria in many patients. Such unexplained hematuria presents a management dilemma. Although most urology specialists/one-stop clinics will discharge these patients, it has been suggested that repeat urinalysis, cytology and blood pressure monitoring is required. Unexplained frank hematuria requires more extensive investigation.

For patients with persistent asymptomatic microhematuria with no etiologic findings or associations, one approach is to evaluate them twice, 6 to 12 months apart, and then only if the amount increases or symptoms appear.

Key points – hematuria

- Blood in the urine can originate from anywhere along the urinary tract and may indicate underlying pathology.
- Dipstick testing is sensitive but does not distinguish between physiological and pathological amounts of blood.
- The most common causes of hematuria are stones, infection, nephritis and prostate enlargement. Malignancy becomes more likely in patients over 50 years of age and who smoke. Some drugs can cause hematuria.
- The morphology of red blood cells may distinguish between glomerular and lower urinary tract causes.
- Investigation of hematuria can be in a 'one stop' clinic with facilities for cytology, ultrasonography and flexible cystoscopy so that diagnosis can be made in one visit.
- Ultrasonography is useful for identifying renal parenchymal disease and urinary tract obstruction. Radiography will identify stones. CT scanning is highly sensitive for detecting stones, renal masses and infections.
- Management depends on the underlying cause identified.
- Unexplained hematuria should be followed up with repeat tests at a later date.

Key references

Grossfeld GD, Wolf JS Jr, Litwan MS et al. Asymptomatic microscopic hematuria in adults: summary of the AUA best practice policy recommendations. *Am Fam Physician* 2001;63:1145–54.

Raghavan D, Bailey M. *Fast Facts: Bladder Cancer*, 2nd edn. Oxford: Health Press, 2006.

Rodgers MA, Hempel S, Aho T et al. Diagnostic tests used in the investigation of adult haematuria. A systematic review. *BJU Int* 2006;98:1154–60.

Rodgers M, Nixon J, Hempel S et al. Diagnostic tests and algorithms used in the investigation of haematuria: systematic reviews and economic evaluation. *Health Technol Assess* 2006;10:xi–259.

Asymptomatic bacteriuria

Asymptomatic bacteriuria refers to the finding of a significant number of bacteria in the urine of a patient but without any of the symptoms of urinary tract infection (UTI). The prevalence varies from 5% of premenopausal women to more than 15% in the elderly; almost 100% of patients with a long-term (longer than 30 days) indwelling urinary catheter are affected.

Because of the increasing problem of bacterial resistance to antibiotics, it is important to rationalize treatment of asymptomatic bacteriuria. The majority of patients will not benefit from antibiotic treatment, and it is thus not indicated. However, it is important to treat asymptomatic infections in a small number of patient groups, as summarized in Table 7.1.

Recurrent urinary tract infection

Recurrent UTI is defined as a UTI followed by a further infection after resolution of the initial bacteriuria. Often this reinfection is caused by repeated contamination of the urinary tract with perineal flora.

Epidemiology. Women are much more susceptible to UTIs than are men; at least 20–30% of women will have a UTI at some time in their life, and 25% of these women will develop recurrent UTI.

TABLE 7.1

Groups in whom treatment of asymptomatic bacteriuria is warranted

- Pregnant women – up to 40% will develop a kidney infection if asymptomatic bacteriuria is left untreated
- Kidney transplant recipients
- Young children with vesico–ureteral reflux
- Patients with infected kidney stones

The bacteria most commonly associated with UTI are *Escherichia coli* (80%) and *Klebsiella* (5%), *Enterobacter* (2%) and *Proteus* (2%) spp. *Staphylococcus saprophyticus* causes 10% of cases of acute cystitis in young women. Anaerobic infections of the urinary tract are rare.

Etiology. Table 7.2 lists the underlying pathologies that should be considered, although it is unlikely that an underlying abnormality will be identified.

The normal estrogenized vaginal flora inhibits the growth of *E. coli* and other Gram-negative fecal flora, possibly through the production of hydrogen peroxide. Alteration of this flora may promote the growth of bacteria that are pathogenic to the urinary tract. Glycogen stores in genital tract epithelial cells are depleted after the menopause, and the environment is less supportive of *Lactobacilli* spp. growth. There is therefore increased colonization of the vagina with *Enterobacter* spp. Vaginal pH increases after the menopause, making these women more prone to UTI.

Symptoms of lower UTI include frequency of micturition, urgency, dysuria and suprapubic discomfort. Women with lower UTI are usually systemically well, but symptoms such as fever, with or without rigors, malaise, nausea and vomiting may occur if the infection ascends. Renal angle pain and tenderness are often predominant

TABLE 7.2

Pathologies that may lead to recurrent urinary tract infection

- Bladder or urethral diverticulum
- Urinary tract calculi
- Bowel fistula (normally secondary to Crohn's disease, diverticulitis or radiation treatment)
- Urethral strictures/any cause of obstruction
- Carcinoma
- Incomplete bladder emptying

features of pyelonephritis. In the elderly patient, mental changes, malaise and confusion may be the only presenting symptoms of a UTI.

Diagnosis. Urinalysis, using dipstick tests for leukocytes and bacterial nitrite production, is quick and easy. A positive dipstick test result has sensitivity in the region of 70% and a specificity of 80% for finding significant pathogens in urine. Microscopy remains the gold standard for the diagnosis of UTI, and urine must be cultured in the presence of antimicrobials to determine sensitivities.

Investigation. The extent to which recurrent UTI should be investigated is controversial; it does, however, make sense to rule out the common pathological abnormalities. It is important to note that UTIs are relatively rare in men and are therefore more likely to have a significant cause than in women.

Tests performed can include an estimation of postvoid residual urine volume, outpatient cystoscopy and imaging of the upper urinary tract, usually with ultrasonography and plain radiography, looking for calculi, evidence of reflux and cortical scarring. However, such investigations will prove negative in the majority of patients, and a degree of clinical discretion is required to prevent the expense and distress caused by overinvestigation, particularly in young women in whom concurrent pathology is unlikely.

Further investigation will depend on clinical factors such as the coexistence of hematuria (see Chapter 6), the severity of symptoms and the presence of atypical organisms such as *P. mirabilis*, which is commonly found in association with stones.

Treatment. Any underlying cause should be treated. Patients who are found to have incomplete bladder emptying, with postvoid residual volumes that are consistently greater than 100 mL, should be taught to double void (Table 7.3). Intermittent self-catheterization (see Chapter 9, pages 102–4) to empty the bladder fully at least once a day should be recommended for patients with large postvoid residual volumes.

TABLE 7.3

Strategies to ensure complete bladder emptying

- Empty your bladder in a relaxed and private place – worry and tension can make bladder emptying harder
- For women: sit comfortably on the toilet seat and relax the pelvic floor muscle to void
- For men: you can stand, but if it seems hard to urinate fully when standing, then you can sit
- Do not push down on your bladder with your hands or stomach to help urinate
- Double voiding can help your bladder empty; here are ways to do it:
  - change the position of your upper body by rocking or leaning forward on the toilet, *or*
  - once you have stopped urinating, stand up, sit back down, lean forward and try to void again, *or*
  - when urinating stops, wait on the toilet for 3 to 5 minutes and then exhale through your mouth only, as if you are blowing through a straw, then try urinating

Urethral dilatation has been a common treatment, particularly in women, but there is little evidence to support its use unless a urethral stricture is present.

In rare cases of vesicoureteric reflux, submucosal injection of collagen or another approved bulking agent in the ureterovesical junction or ureteric reimplantation may be indicated to protect the kidneys from damage.

The majority of investigations, however, will be normal, and treatment should be on the basis of symptoms.

Adequate fluid intake (at least 2 liters/day) will help to maintain a good urine output to flush pathogens away. Patients should void frequently and completely, and women should be advised to void before bed and after sexual intercourse.

Cranberries contain substances such as fructose that inhibit the adherence of some bacteria (e.g. *E. coli*) to uroepithelial cells.

Cranberries are thought to contain a substance that can reduce the incidence of UTIs by changing the surface properties of *E. coli*, preventing it from adhering to the wall of the bladder. A Cochrane review found that cranberry products significantly reduced the incidence of UTIs over 12 months. Recommendations are for cranberry tablets, 1 tablet (300–400 mg) twice daily or unsweetened juice (~250 mL or 8 oz) three times daily.

Antibiotic treatment is recommended for patients with recurrent UTIs. Acute infections should be treated with a short course of an appropriate antibiotic, the type depending on local resistance. The majority of uncomplicated lower UTIs respond to a 3-day course of trimethoprim or a 7-day course of amoxicillin or nitrofurantoin. However, urine culture before treatment is important, given the widespread resistance to antibiotics. Alternative antibiotics for resistant organisms include co-amoxiclav, oral cephalosporins or a quinolone.

Antibiotic prophylaxis. A continuous regimen of low-dose antibiotics can be used as prophylaxis against further infections in selected patients. At low doses, an adequate concentration of antibiotic will be achieved in the urine but with little effect on the fecal and vaginal flora, thereby preventing the development of resistant strains and complications related to the reduction of normal flora, such as genital *Candida* spp. infections. A single antibiotic can be used: trimethoprim, cefalexin and nitrofurantoin are commonly recommended. These remain effective in the long term despite continued use. Significant resistance does not develop, and adverse effects are rare. Some clinicians recommend a 3-monthly rotating regimen of different antimicrobials to minimize any small chance of promoting resistant strains.

Prophylactic antibiotic use reduces the frequency of infections by 95%, to a mean of fewer than 0.2 infections per year. Breakthrough infections should be treated with full doses of appropriate antibiotics.

Consideration should be given to stopping the prophylactic regimen after 6–12 months to see if the frequency of infections has altered. However, some patients may need to continue daily prophylaxis for life. An alternative to prophylaxis is to allow patients to self-medicate. Patients are provided with 3 days' full-dose antibiotic treatment to take when they experience the symptoms of acute cystitis; the symptoms of UTIs can be accurately identified by 85% of women. Postcoital antibiotics will be beneficial for some women if sexual intercourse appears to be the sole predisposing factor.

Suppressing UTI in patients with bacterial colonization can be done using methenamine hippurate, a urinary antiseptic that releases formaldehyde and keeps colony counts low. The dosage is 1 g combined with vitamin C, 1 g, twice daily.

Vaginal estrogen. There is some evidence that vaginal estrogen is beneficial in postmenopausal women with recurrent UTIs. It increases the cellular glycogen concentration and encourages recolonization with *Lactobacilli* spp., thus reducing the vaginal pH and therefore the concentration of pathogenic bacteria. Vaginal estrogens can be delivered locally via creams, tablets and a ring.

Bladder pain syndrome and interstitial cystitis

Bladder pain syndrome (BPS) and interstitial cystitis (IC) are described in the American Urological Association IC/BPS guideline as a condition in which a patient experiences an unpleasant sensation (pain, pressure, discomfort) perceived to be related to the urinary bladder, associated with lower urinary tract symptoms of more than 6 weeks' duration, in the absence of infection or other identifiable causes. BPS is the encompassing term. The diagnosis of IC is confined to patients with painful bladder symptoms who have characteristic cystoscopic and histological features.

Epidemiology. There is no real agreement as to the true incidence of BPS or IC, as there are no formalized diagnostic criteria. Estimates of the incidence of the latter vary from 8 to 1600 per 100 000.

It is commonly accepted that IC predominates in women. Estimates of population prevalence indicate male-to-female ratios of 1:4.5 to 1:9, although few studies have included enough men to show whether there are true sex differences.

Etiology. Despite extensive scientific effort, the precise etiology of BPS and IC has yet to be explained. The initial descriptions of IC by Guy

85

Hunner in 1918 included loss of epithelium, with the underlying mucosa showing granulation tissue, increased capillaries, edema and chronic inflammatory cells, also involving the muscle coat and thickened peritoneum over the diseased area. Precisely what causes these changes is not known, and no causal agent has been found. These changes are generally considered to be late changes, and many patients with BPS/IC have no specific cystoscopic findings.

Symptoms. The diagnosis of BPS/IC is based clinically on symptoms of urinary frequency, urgency and pain. Pain is an essential component of both conditions and is traditionally described as increasing pain on bladder filling that is relieved by voiding. It is recognized that pain may present as bladder, urethral, vaginal, vulval, rectal or pelvic pain, and it may be suprapubic, urethral, perineal or a combination. There are no criteria for the nature or location of the pain except that it must be chronic and have no other obvious cause.

Diagnosis of BPS or IC requires the exclusion of other causes of the bladder symptoms, such as infection, malignancy, radiation or drug-induced cystitis.

Cystoscopy and biopsy. The classic cystoscopic picture of IC is one of punctate petechial hemorrhages observed on second-look cystoscopy after cystodistension to 70–80 cmH$_2$O for 1–3 minutes. This needs to be carried out under general anesthesia; outpatient flexible cystoscopy is inadequate to make this diagnosis. These cystoscopic findings are not necessarily diagnostic, however, as not all patients with petechial hemorrhages have IC, and vice versa.

Bladder biopsy may show changes such as infiltration with inflammatory cells in all or specific parts of the bladder wall, but more commonly shows no characteristic pattern of inflammation.

There is some disagreement about the role of cystoscopy and bladder biopsy in the diagnosis of IC. Some clinicians will diagnose IC in a patient who has a 3-month history of urinary urgency and frequency, bladder pain relieved by voiding and a negative urinary culture and cytology, whereas others will diagnose the condition only if the characteristic cystoscopic findings are present, preferably with histological confirmation. Biopsy is clinically indicated only if there is a suspicion of malignancy or as part of a clinical protocol.

Management. Once the diagnosis of BPS/IC is made, the next decision is whether to initiate treatment or to consider a course of 'watchful waiting'. The natural history of the disorder is not fully understood, and the proportion of patients whose symptoms will resolve spontaneously is not known. Treatment is not always necessary if a patient's symptoms are tolerable and do not impact significantly on quality of life; there are few data to show that treatment will significantly alter the natural history of the disorder. However, patients who present with BPS/IC should receive behavior modification treatment, as described in Table 7.4.

Education and empowerment have important roles, and patients are reassured to know that their symptoms are part of a recognized

TABLE 7.4

Behavior modification and self-care practices for bladder pain syndrome/interstitial cystitis

- Dietary training: identification and avoidance of dietary 'triggers' (e.g. acidic drinks, spicy foods, caffeine, alcohol)
- Altering the concentration and/or volume of urine, either by fluid restriction or additional hydration
- Application of local heat over the bladder or perineum
- Adjustment of urinary pH with certain products (e.g. pyridium or calcium glycerophosphate, which may have additional symptom-alleviating effects)
- Techniques applied to trigger points and areas of hypersensitivity (e.g. application of heat or cold)
- Strategies to manage flare-ups (e.g. meditation, imagery)
- Pelvic floor muscle relaxation
- Bladder training with urge suppression
- Manual physical therapy

TABLE 7.5

**Other treatment options for bladder pain syndrome/
interstitial cystitis***

- Pharmacological treatment
  - tricyclic antidepressants (see Table 7.6)
  - analgesics
  - sodium pentosan polysulfate
  - intravesical injection of clorpactin, dimethyl sulfoxide, heparin, hyaluronic acid, sodium pentosan polysulfate
- Invasive treatment (if all else fails and symptoms are debilitating)
  - sacral nerve stimulation (see Chapter 4, pages 58–60)
  - augmentation cystoplasty (rarely)

*If management is chosen over watchful waiting.

syndrome that affects many people. Options for treatment are summarized in Tables 7.4 and 7.5.

Dietary advice. Many patients find that BPS/IC seems to be affected by particular foods, mostly 'acidic' drinks, spicy foods, caffeine and alcohol. A wide variety of foods has been implicated and special diets for patients with BPS/IC are provided in patient information. Not all foods affect all patients in the same way so it is important to advise patients to avoid only those foods that affect them.

Behavioral changes. Modifying certain behaviors can improve symptoms in some IC/BPS patients and can reduce the frequency of voiding.

Oral treatments. The effects of therapy are difficult to evaluate, given the uncertain natural history of the condition and the fact that the condition tends to vary in severity. The following drugs have been reported to be beneficial.

Tricyclic antidepressants used in the treatment of BPS/IC are listed in Table 7.6. Amitriptyline is commonly used for its analgesic properties, although the mechanism of action is not known. It has been used in the treatment of BPS/IC and is useful in the management

TABLE 7.6

Tricyclic antidepressants used to treat interstitial cystitis

- Amitriptyline
- Imipramine
- Nortriptyline
- Desipramine
- Doxepin

of pain at a titrated dose of up to 75 mg daily. Its effectiveness is limited by side effects of drowsiness, fatigue, weight gain and dry mouth – approximately one-third of patients cannot tolerate amitriptyline.

Analgesics. The appropriate long-term use of analgesics plays an integral role in the conservative management of BPS/IC. Most patients can be helped by using medications used for chronic neuropathic pain syndromes, including antidepressants, anticonvulsants and opioids (see *Fast Facts: Chronic and Cancer Pain*). Many non-steroidal anti-inflammatory drugs are useful, and there is interest in the use of cyclooxygenase-2 inhibitors.

Antibiotics. There is currently no role for antibiotics in the management of BPS/IC in the absence of a laboratory-proven UTI.

Hydroxyzine is a histamine H_1 receptor antagonist that inhibits bladder mast-cell activation. It has been reported to reduce frequency, nocturia and pain in a small proportion of patients, but efficacy was not demonstrated in a double-blind randomized controlled trial.

Sodium pentosan polysulfate is a heparin analog available in an oral formulation, 3–6% of which is excreted into the urine. Although this is the only oral agent approved for the treatment of IC, expert opinion of its efficacy is divided. As a sulfated mucopolysaccharide, sodium pentosan polysulfate is hypothesized to repair defects in the glycoaminoglycan layer of the epithelial permeability barrier, which are thought to contribute to the pathogenesis of IC. It has been reported by advocates as beneficial in that it reduces the symptoms of IC to a modestly greater extent than placebo. A 3–6-month course is needed to demonstrate an effect; the dose is 100 mg three times a day. Sodium pentosan polysulfate is well tolerated and produces few side effects.

Intravesical therapy. Several drugs are available for intravesical therapy of BPS/IC. These include clorpactin, dimethyl sulfoxide (DMSO), heparin, lidocaine, hyaluronic acid and sodium pentosan polysulfate.

The intravesical route of administration provides high local drug concentrations in the bladder, avoids systemic side effects and eliminates the problem of low levels of urinary excretion with orally administered agents. Agents are given weekly or every 2 weeks for a total of 4–8 treatments. Some clinicians continue with maintenance instillations on a monthly basis. Long-term remission will be achieved in some patients with this approach, but in most the condition will relapse eventually and require additional treatments.

Treatment with intravesical agents does not require anesthesia or hospital admission, and some patients can be taught to self-administer the drugs.

Invasive treatment should be reserved for patients with debilitating symptoms in whom conservative treatments have failed.

Sacral nerve stimulation (see Figure 4.2 and pages 58–60) involves the percutaneous stimulation of the S3 or S4 nerve root. Initially it is carried out with a temporary stimulator; a permanent implant can be inserted if the patient responds. It may be helpful for the symptoms of urgency and frequency but does not appear to improve pain associated with BPS/IC.

Augmentation cystoplasty was used for refractory bladder pain for many years but is rarely used nowadays. The procedure involves using a segment of bowel to enlarge the bladder and has been performed with or without excision of the diseased bladder segment. However, results are generally poor for classic BPS/IC.

Key points – urinary tract infections and cystitis

- Recurrent urinary tract infection (UTI) is defined as a further UTI after resolution of initial bacteriuria.
- At least 20–30% of women will have a UTI at some time, 25% of whom will develop recurrent UTI. UTIs are relatively rare in men and are more likely to have a significant cause than in women.
- Urinalysis is quick and easy. A positive test should be followed up by microscopy, and the urine cultured to determine antimicrobial sensitivity.
- Treatment of UTIs is largely on the basis of symptoms and any underlying identified cause.
- Antibiotic treatment is recommended for recurrent UTI; prophylactic antibiotics and self-medication should also be considered.
- Bladder pain syndrome (BPS) is characterized by suprapubic pain relating to bladder filling, accompanied by other symptoms such as frequency, in the absence of a proven UTI or other pathology. The diagnosis of interstitial cystitis (IC) is confined to patients with bladder pain symptoms with characteristic cytoscopic and histological features.
- The etiology of BPS/IC is largely unknown.
- The roles of cystoscopy and bladder biopsy in the diagnosis of BPS/IC are controversial.
- Management of BPS/IC is largely conservative, and includes dietary advice, behavioral therapies, and oral and intravesical medication.

Key references

Albert X, Huertas I, Pereiró, II et al. Antibiotics for preventing recurrent urinary tract infection in non-pregnant women. *Cochrane Database Syst Rev* 2004(3): CD001209.

Anonymous. Screening for asymptomatic bacteriuria in adults: U.S. Preventive Services Task Force reaffirmation recommendation statement. *Ann Intern Med* 2008;149:43–7.

Cousins MJ, Gallagher RM. *Fast Facts: Chronic and Cancer Pain, 2nd edn.* Oxford: Health Press, 2011.

Franco AV. Recurrent urinary tract infections. *Best Pract Res Clin Obstet Gynaecol* 2005;19:861–73.

Hanno PM. Painful bladder syndrome / interstitial cystitis and related disorders. In: Wein AJ, Kavoussi LR, Novick AC et al., eds. *Campbell-Walsh Urology.* Philadelphia: Elsevier/Saunders, 2007:330–70.

Hanno PM, Burks DA, Clemens JQ et al. AUA guideline for the diagnosis and treatment of interstitial cystitis/bladder pain syndrome. *J Urol* 2011;185:2162–70.

Jepson RG, Craig JC. Cranberries for preventing urinary tract infections. *Cochrane Database Syst Rev* 2008(1):CD001321.

Moldwin RM, Evans RJ, Stanford EJ, Rosenberg MT. Rational approaches to the treatment of patients with interstitial cystitis. *Urology* 2007;69:73–81.

Rosenberg MT, Newman DK, Page SA. Interstitial cystitis/painful bladder syndrome: symptom recognition is key to early identification, treatment. *Cleve Clin J Med* 2007;74 Suppl 3:S54–62.

Primary nocturnal enufresis

Nocturnal enuresis is the involuntary passage of urine during sleep in children aged 5 years old and above. Primary nocturnal enuresis is urinary incontinence that occurs during sleep in a child who has never regularly been dry at night. It is often referred to as 'bed-wetting' and is a common condition that can cause difficulty for both child and family. Nocturnal enuresis occurs in approximately 20% of 5-year-olds, 10% of 10-year-olds and 1% of 15-year-olds. It is more prevalent among boys than girls.

The majority of children affected are fully continent during the day. The condition is usually self-limiting and children generally become dry at night spontaneously as they get older.

Etiology. Nocturnal enuresis has a number of different etiologies (Table 8.1). If nocturnal enuresis persists beyond 9 years of age, the child should undergo an evaluation.

Investigations. A comprehensive urologic history should be taken to exclude any associated conditions that may require treatment. Physical examination should be carried out, although abnormalities are unlikely to be detected. The specific gravity of an early-morning urine sample should be measured to identify those who may benefit from antidiuretic hormone (ADH; desmopressin) treatment.

A frequency/volume bladder record (see pages 18–20 and Figure 2.3) is one of the most important tools in the investigation and management of primary nocturnal enuresis. It will provide detailed information about fluid intake and voided volumes during the day and episodes of bed-wetting during the night. It can be used to assess the severity of the problem and also provides a baseline against which the effects of treatment can be measured.

Renal ultrasound and uroflowmetry are required only when symptoms are suggestive of urinary tract dysfunction. Urodynamic

TABLE 8.1

Potential etiologies of nocturnal enuresis

- High fluid intake in association with deep sleeping
- Small bladder capacity
- Constipation
- Reduced urine osmolarity decreases nocturnal secretion of antidiuretic hormone (ADH; desmopressin), leading to increased night-time urine production
- Detrusor overactivity, seen in 25% of children with nocturnal enuresis with no daytime symptoms
- Upper airway obstruction is associated with nocturnal enuresis; the condition improves with treatment such as tonsillectomy
- Family history, noted in 65–77% of children with nocturnal enuresis
- Psychological factors, possibly (some disagreement)

studies should be reserved for the child with diurnal symptoms that fail to respond to conventional treatments.

Treatment. Many different treatments have been tried for nocturnal enuresis, with varying degrees of success. The success rates of common treatments are shown in Table 8.2.

Reassurance. The majority of children will grow out of bed-wetting, and reassurance may be all that is necessary. However, most parents and children ask for treatment because of the inconvenience and social difficulty that bed-wetting causes.

Changes in fluid intake and therefore output are the simplest means of improving the condition; keeping a diary is important to record improvements. It is important not to set a high and unattainable goal too early or the child will lose interest. Although parents are often tempted to control evening drinking, this may be counterproductive because concentrated urine can irritate the bladder.

Behavioral therapy. If the child wets the bed at a particular time of night, a waking regimen may be of benefit. Behavioral therapy

TABLE 8.2

Efficacy of common treatments for nocturnal enuresis

Treatment	Efficacy
Observation only	• 6% continent at 6 months; 16% at 1 year
Drug therapy	
ADH (desmopressin)	• Improvement in 79% of patients at 1 year; 50% long-term improvement
	• 68% continent at 6 months; 10% continent at 1 year
	• 81% improved by 12 weeks
	• 48% dry and 22% improved
Amitriptyline	• Effective at reducing number of wet nights
Imipramine	• 36% continent at 6 months; 16% at 1 year; 73% improved
Behavioral interventions	
Alarms and sensors	• 84% dry
	• 63% continent at 6 months; 56% at 1 year
Waking schedule and full-spectrum home training	• 76% dry
Motivation counseling	• 23% cure rate (many more helped)
Acupuncture	• 55% effective at 1 year; 40% long-term improvement
Combination – drugs	• May produce a complementary benefit if combined with alarms

ADH, antidiuretic hormone.

and biofeedback are useful non-pharmacological treatments. Alarms that sense bed-wetting (called moisture-sensing alarms) can be used from the age of 7 years, but become most effective after the age of

10 years when the child is able to take responsibility for him- or herself.

Pharmacological treatment. Antimuscarinic drugs (see Table 4.3, page 55) can be beneficial. ADH (desmopressin) will reduce nocturnal urine output and provide dry nights, but is not recommended for continuous long-term use because of alterations in serum electrolytes, specifically hyponatremia. However, it can be useful if a child is sleeping away from home.

Persistence into adolescence. Only 1% of adolescents (by age 15 years) still experience nocturnal enuresis, and 15% of these become dry with each subsequent year. By 15 years of age, urodynamic studies should be performed to check for abnormalities in detrusor function, the commonest of these being detrusor overactivity. Occult neurological dysfunction may be responsible for enuresis in a small number of patients. After the age of 18 years, patients with persistent enuresis due to detrusor overactivity that does not respond to non-surgical treatment could be offered treatment with botulinum toxin or bladder augmentation (see Chapter 4, pages 57–8 and 60, respectively).

Nocturia and nocturnal polyuria

Nocturia is defined as waking from sleep once or more to void. The 'official' definition by the International Continence Society specifies that each void is preceded and followed by sleep. The threshold for bother is debatable: either two or three times. Prevalence estimates (referring to two or more episodes) are 2–17% in men aged 20–40 years, 4–18% in women aged 20–40 years, 29–59% in men over the age of 70, and 28–62% in women over 70. Nocturia may be associated with the following negative impacts: reduced quality of life and productivity; increased incidence of falls and fractures (particularly among the elderly); mood disturbances; increased daytime fatigue; and decreased alertness. The pathophysiology is shown in Figure 8.1

Nocturnal polyuria is defined as nocturnal urine output of more than 20% of the daily total in young adults and more than 33% in older adults. Nocturnal polyuria is a contributory factor in up to 83% of patients with nocturia. Overactive bladder is estimated to be a

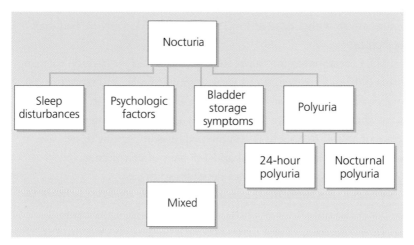

Figure 8.1 The pathophysiology of nocturia. After Wein et al., 2002.

contributing factor in 17–33%, and the incidence of nocturia in patients with overactive bladder is estimated to range from 50–80%.

Investigation. The frequency/volume bladder record (see pages 18–20 and Figure 2.3) is the most useful tool for investigating nocturia: it will provide information about the number of night-time voids and fluid intake, particularly in the evening and night.

Urodynamic studies can be carried out to identify detrusor overactivity. If congestive cardiac failure is suspected, the appropriate investigations and referral should be made.

Treatment of nocturia should be on the basis of identified underlying causes. Simple measures can be implemented, such as reducing evening and nighttime fluid intake. The frail elderly should be provided with a bedside commode or urinal, to minimize the risk of falls while going to the bathroom. An upright rail fixed to the bed to facilitate getting out safely is also important. Patients who have peripheral edema and vascular insufficiency may benefit from the use of support stockings during the day, leg elevation in the afternoon and reduction in salt intake. Treatment of sleep apnea can improve nocturia.

Pharmacological treatment aims to shift the diuresis to the daytime. Reducing the volume overload associated with congestive

97

heart failure with a dose of loop diuretic 6–8 hours before bed may be helpful.

ADH (desmopressin) has been used successfully to reduce nocturnal urine output. However, it can cause hyponatremia, and there is a risk of exacerbating congestive cardiac failure, particularly in the elderly; some therefore consider it not generally suitable for patients over 65 years of age. If treatment is commenced, it is important to measure serum electrolytes beforehand and 1–3 days after commencing treatment, as hyponatremia can develop rapidly.

A trial of antimuscarinic agent (see Table 4.3, page 55) is likely to be beneficial only if the nocturia is associated with significant nocturnal detrusor overactivity. Having a patient take the drug at bedtime may help to decrease nocturia.

Key points – nocturnal symptoms

- Primary nocturnal enuresis is urinary incontinence that occurs at night in a child who has never been regularly dry at night.
- It is a relatively common condition, but generally resolves spontaneously and rarely persists into adolescence.
- The frequency/volume bladder record is the most useful investigative tool for primary nocturnal enuresis and also helps in monitoring treatment.
- Treatment of primary nocturnal enuresis is rarely required, but can include modification of fluid intake, behavioral treatments and occasional use of ADH (desmopressin).
- Nocturia – defined as waking from sleep to void – has a significant impact on quality of life and is a major cause of falls in the elderly.
- Treatment of nocturia is largely on the basis of the underlying cause. Loop diuretics in the afternoon may be useful if nocturia is related to congestive heart failure. ADH should be used with caution, as it can cause rapid hyponatremia. Antimuscarinics may prove useful only in patients with severe nocturnal detrusor overactivity.

Key references

Berry AK. Helping children with nocturnal enuresis: the wait-and-see approach may not be in anyone's best interest. *Am J Nurs* 2006; 106:56–63.

Burgio KL, Johnson TM, 2nd, Goode PS et al. Prevalence and correlates of nocturia in community-dwelling older adults. *J Am Geriatr Soc* 2010;58:861–6.

Glazener CM, Evans JH. Simple behavioural and physical interventions for nocturnal enuresis in children. *Cochrane Database Syst Rev* 2004(2):CD003637.

Glazener CM, Evans JH. Desmopressin for nocturnal enuresis in children. *Cochrane Database Syst Rev* 2002(3):CD002112.

Glazener CM, Evans JH, Peto RE. Drugs for nocturnal enuresis in children (other than desmopressin and tricyclics). *Cochrane Database Syst Rev* 2003(4):CD002238.

Lyon C, Schnall J. What is the best treatment for nocturnal enuresis in children? *J Fam Pract* 2005;54:905–6.

Tikkinen KA, Auvinen A, Johnson TM, 2nd et al. A systematic evaluation of factors associated with nocturia–the population-based FINNO study. *Am J Epidemiol* 2009;170:361–8.

Van Kerrebroeck P, Abrams P, Chaikin D et al. The standardization of terminology in nocturia: report from the standardization subcommittee of the International Continence Society. *BJU Int* 2002;90(suppl 3):11–15.

Vaughan CP, Brown CJ, Goode PS et al. The association of nocturia with incident falls in an elderly community-dwelling cohort. *Int J Clin Pract* 2010;64:577–83.

Wein A, Lose GR, Fonda D. Nocturia in men, women and the elderly: a practical approach. *BJU Int* 2002;90(suppl 3):28–31.

Weiss JP, Blaivas JG, Bliwise DL et al. The evaluation and treatment of nocturia: a consensus statement. *BJU Int* 2011;108:6–21.

Most neurological diseases that affect the spinal cord and some that affect the brain will cause bladder dysfunction, which, if untreated, may lead to incontinence. Neuropathic bladder dysfunction (also referred to as neurogenic bladder) can be divided into three types of disorder according to the site of the lesion: suprapontine, suprasacral spinal and peripheral. Urodynamic investigation is required to distinguish between the different types of filling/storage and voiding dysfunction that may result.

Lesion types

Suprapontine lesions tend to lead to detrusor overactivity, although coordinated sphincter function is preserved. These lesions can therefore result in frequency, urgency and urgency incontinence. The principal causes of suprapontine lesions are dementia, cerebrovascular accident, closed head injury and Parkinson's disease.

Suprasacral spinal lesions that interfere with reflex control of the bladder from the higher centers will produce detrusor overactivity. This is seen in many patients with neurological bladder dysfunction and is characterized by spontaneous involuntary detrusor contractions, with or without the sensation of urgency, leading to urinary incontinence. Detrusor overactivity may be associated with non-coordination of the external urethral sphincter, which contracts during detrusor contraction, termed detrusor–sphincter dyssynergia (DSD). This causes hypertrophy of detrusor smooth muscle (trabeculation) as a result of the frequent, high-pressure, sustained detrusor contractions in the presence of obstruction. Patients with detrusor overactivity and DSD not only experience urinary incontinence but may also develop long-term effects of high intravesical pressures, giving rise to ureteric reflux or obstruction, or both, and resulting in renal damage and failure.

The causes of suprasacral spinal lesions include multiple sclerosis, spinal cord injury and infections (e.g. transverse myelitis), spina bifida and tumors that affect the suprasacral spinal cord.

Peripheral lesions. Injury or disease that affects the nerve roots or peripheral nerves (spinal trauma, myelomeningocele, pelvic surgery, diabetes mellitus) causes bladder areflexia or acontractility and, as a result, the bladder fails to empty unless voiding is assisted by straining. In patients with such lesions, the external urethral sphincter may fail to relax (isolated distal sphincter obstruction) and may also be weakened, giving rise to stress incontinence.

Diagnosis

The diagnosis of neuropathic bladder disorders requires an understanding of the underlying neurological abnormality, which will be apparent in most patients. However, some patients will present with the symptoms of a neuropathic bladder but with no overt neurological cause. In this situation, it is important to consider the possibility of an undiagnosed neurological condition such as multiple sclerosis or spinal cord lesion, as neuropathic bladder may be the presenting symptom. In patients with cervical lesions, especially those with complete spinal cord transection, it may be difficult to assess symptoms as many will be atypical or unconscious rather than the classic 'urge' type symptoms.

Patients with acontractile bladders tend to leak urine as a result of retention with overflow or in association with sphincter weakness.

Apart from neurological examination, urodynamic investigation is essential to make an appropriate diagnosis and provide treatment.

Management

The aim of treating the neuropathic bladder is to enable low-pressure storage of urine and bladder emptying without obstruction. Treatment of detrusor overactivity is therefore focused on reducing detrusor muscle contractions and/or reducing the effect of DSD, if present, by lowering the resistance of the external urethral sphincter.

Control of detrusor overactivity with antimuscarinic drugs or surgery is described in Chapter 4 (pages 54–7 and 60, respectively). If oral therapy cannot be tolerated, intravesical agents such as botulinum toxin or oxybutynin may be used.

Reducing resistance in the external urethral sphincter can be achieved by a number of methods: sphincterotomy, sphincter stenting or injection of botulinum toxin. These procedures are only suitable for men, who should be counseled about the risk of continuous incontinence afterwards.

In women, a reduction in detrusor contractility will often lead to urinary retention, and intermittent self-catheterization may be necessary to drain the bladder fully (see below).

Sphincter weakness or stress incontinence, which accompanies neurological bladder dysfunction, may be resolved by procedures to enhance the bladder outlet (see Chapter 3, pages 41–7).

Catheterization. Despite these measures, some patients will continue to have problems with DSD and will require catheterization to empty the bladder and prevent the long-term complications associated with the condition. The options for these patients are intermittent self-catheterization, or long-term indwelling catheterization with a urethral or suprapubic catheter.

Intermittent self-catheterization (ISC) is useful in any condition in which bladder emptying is impaired in association with adequate outlet resistance. Many patients catheterize themselves on a regular basis throughout the day (and night) to ensure bladder emptying. (Figure 9.1) In patients with neuropathic bladder, the number of catheterizations required will depend on factors such as fluid intake, ambient temperature, bladder capacity and social factors; most patients need to catheterize four or five times each day. If possible, the patient should void prior to catheterization.

For self-catheterization to be successful in patients with neuropathic bladder dysfunction, the bladder must be able to store urine adequately without leaking, a condition that can be facilitated through

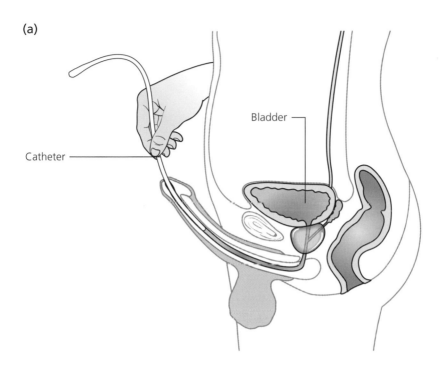

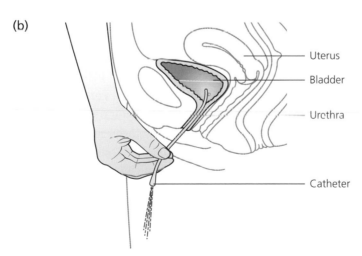

Figure 9.1 Self-catheterization in (a) men, and (b) women. Redrawn with permission from Diane K Newman.

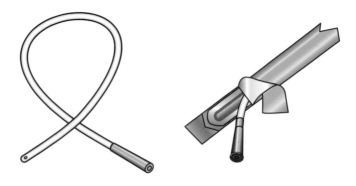

Figure 9.2 Examples of catheters used for intermittent self-catheterization.

the use of antimuscarinic medication (see Table 4.3, page 55).
The patient must be physically able and motivated to perform
catheterization, or a caregiver must be able to do it for them. Patients
and caregivers need access to healthcare professionals who can teach
them the technique and provide adequate support and appropriate
catheters. Examples of catheters used for ISC are shown in Figure 9.2.

Long-term indwelling catheterization (Figure 9.3) is usually a last
resort when all other treatments have failed. However, it may
occasionally be used for shorter periods (< 30 days) if patients are
undecided about their preferred management option. For long-term
catheterization, the suprapubic catheter avoids urethral damage, and is
more comfortable and better tolerated than a catheter inserted via the
urethra. It is also easier to change on a regular basis and causes less
discomfort than may be experienced when changing a urethral
catheter. If dislodged inadvertently, the tract may close and so rapid
replacement is desirable, however.

Any indwelling catheter left in place for a long period of time has
the potential for significant complications (e.g. catheter-associated
urinary tract infection [UTI], urethral erosion and bladder stones).

Insertion of a suprapubic catheter should be carried out under
ultrasound or cystoscopic guidance, as there is a risk of bowel trauma

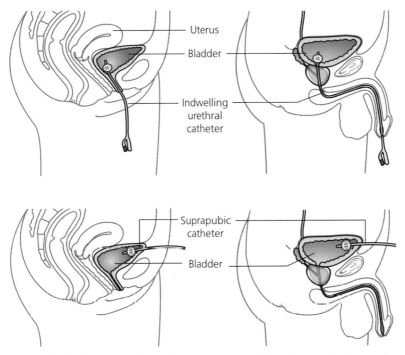

Figure 9.3 Positioning of indwelling and suprapubic catheters in men and women.

from incorrect placement of the catheter. Mortality associated with insertion has been reported as being up to 2%.

Catheter problems. If a suprapubic catheter falls out it is important that it is replaced quickly, ideally immediately. The tract may start to close quickly, and after 2 hours it may be impossible to reinsert the catheter without dilatation of the tract. It is therefore essential that the patient is transferred to hospital immediately if no one is available to insert a replacement catheter. Patients should keep a spare catheter at home in case problems arise.

Catheter blockage is a common problem, usually occurring as a result of the formation of biofilms – collections of microorganisms that coat catheter surfaces leading to encrustation and blockage. Some patients are more prone to catheter blockage than others. If blockage occurs on a regular basis, imaging and/or cystoscopy should be performed to look for bladder calculi or other abnormalities. If

105

investigation suggests calculi, cystoscopy should be performed and the stones removed. Patients who frequently have blocked catheters should be managed with high fluid intake, more regular catheter changes and changing to different catheter material. Other problems seen with urethral or suprapubic indwelling catheters include catheter-associated UTIs, bypassing of urine around the catheter, pain and discomfort, bladder stones and hematuria.

Catheter changes. In general, most indwelling catheters need to be changed every 4–6 weeks. The catheter should be changed by an appropriately trained person, who can be a doctor, nurse, caregiver, relative or the patient.

Follow-up. All patients with spinal cord injury and bladder dysfunction are susceptible to renal damage if the intravesical pressure is not adequately controlled. Yearly follow-up with at least ultrasonography of the upper urinary tracts and measurement of serum creatinine is therefore essential. There is a risk of malignancy with indwelling catheters, especially after lengthy periods of time, although there is no agreement on the magnitude of risk. Many, therefore, feel such patients should undergo yearly cystoscopies and bladder washes for cytology.

Key points – neuropathic bladder dysfunction

- Neuropathic bladder dysfunction can be classified according to the site of the lesion as suprapontine, suprasacral spinal or peripheral.
- Suprapontine lesions are largely associated with Parkinson's disease, dementia and cerebrovascular accident. They usually lead to detrusor overactivity but coordinated sphincter function is preserved.
- Suprasacral spinal lesions are associated with spinal cord injury, spina bifida and tumors, and interfere with the reflex control of the bladder from higher centers, resulting in detrusor overactivity and detrusor–sphincter dyssynergia. Increased intravesical pressure can damage the ureters and, ultimately, the kidneys.
- Peripheral lesions affecting the nerve roots cause bladder areflexia or acontractility, such that the bladder fails to empty without straining. Sphincteric weakness may also contribute to incontinence.
- Management of detrusor overactivity aims to enable low-pressure storage of urine and bladder emptying without obstruction, achieved by antimuscarinic drugs, injection of botulinum toxin or surgery.
- Some patients require catheterization to ensure bladder emptying. Options are intermittent self-catheterization, if the bladder can store urine adequately without leaking (often achieved with antimuscarinic drugs), or a urethral or suprapubic indwelling catheter.

Key references

Bray L, Sanders C. Teaching children and young people intermittent self-catheterization. *Urol Nurs* 2007;27:203–9.

Consortium for Spinal Cord Medicine. Bladder management for adults with spinal cord injury: a clinical practice guideline for health-care providers. *J Spinal Cord Med* 2006;29:527–73.

Newman DK. The indwelling urinary catheter: principles for best practice. *J Wound Ostomy Continence Nurs* 2007;34:655–61.

Newman DK, Willson M. Review of intermittent catheterization and current best practices. *Urologic Nursing* 2011;31:12–29.

Rapidi CA, Panourias IG, Petropoulou K, Sakas DE. Management and rehabilitation of neuropathic bladder in patients with spinal cord lesion. *Acta Neurochir Suppl* 2007;97:307–14.

Samson G, Cardenas DD. Neurogenic bladder in spinal cord injury. *Phys Med Rehabil Clin N Am* 2007;18:255–74.

Stohrer M, Blok B, Castro-Diaz D et al. EAU guidelines on neurogenic lower urinary tract dysfunction. *Eur Urol* 2009;56:81–8.

Wein AJ. Lower urinary tract dysfunction in neurologic injury and disease. In: Wein AJ, Kavoussi LR, Novick AC et al., eds. *Campbell-Walsh Urology*. Philadelphia: Elsevier/Saunders, 2007:2011–45.

The elderly

Lower urinary tract symptoms become more prevalent with age. Management of the symptoms can be challenging, as the elderly are less likely to tolerate surgical or pharmaceutical treatments, and their symptoms are often secondary to multiple causes.

The approach to treatment of these symptoms in the elderly is similar to that in younger people, as the underlying pathophysiology of bladder disorders, such as incontinence and overactive bladder (OAB) does not differ markedly. It is important to rule out or treat constipation and urinary tract infection (UTI) and discontinue inappropriate medication before embarking on extensive investigation.

Urinary incontinence is a frequent cause of institutionalization in the elderly. The common causes of incontinence are similar to those found in younger people, namely bladder overactivity and sphincter weakness, but the effects of aging on the nervous system and the lower urinary tract exacerbate the symptoms.

As in younger people, it is appropriate to determine the cause of incontinence and it is feasible to correct both bladder overactivity and sphincter weakness.

Investigation. Finding the cause of urinary incontinence is more important in the elderly than in younger patients. The elderly are more likely to have multiple coexisting symptoms and may have multiple pathologies to account for them. In addition, the elderly are less likely to tolerate the adverse effects of antimuscarinic medications. Empirical treatment based on symptoms and a frequency/volume bladder record can be unsatisfactory.

Investigation may involve urodynamic investigation, the indications for which are outlined in Chapter 2 (see page 23). Cystometry is well tolerated in the elderly. If cystometry is performed, prophylactic antibiotics should be considered, particularly in patients susceptible to UTIs.

Treatment. If detrusor overactivity is identified, behavioral therapy and antimuscarinic medication can be commenced, taking into account other medications the patient is taking that may cause interactions, such as antidepressants. Treatment should be started with a low dose and the dose increased gradually until the required benefits are obtained with the minimum of adverse effects. Detrusor contractility decreases with age and therefore the incidence of urinary retention with antimuscarinic medications may be higher in the elderly. Also, in the elderly patient, antimuscarinic drugs may be more likely to cause drowsiness and cognitive impairment.

In women, urethral hypermobility becomes a less prevalent cause of urinary stress incontinence with age as vaginal mobility reduces with postmenopausal atrophy. This means that stress incontinence is far more likely to have a significant component of intrinsic sphincter deficiency in these patients, and treatment should be tailored accordingly.

Surgery for stress incontinence is possible in the elderly but general anesthesia and major abdominal surgery are best avoided. Urethral injection therapy or minimally invasive sling insertion under local or regional anesthesia (as described in Chapter 3) are well tolerated.

The risk of postoperative urinary retention is relatively high in the elderly because of their reduced detrusor contractility. Retention is also more difficult to manage, as intermittent self-catheterization can be difficult to perform in those with poor eyesight and reduced manual dexterity.

Urethral injection therapy is preferred in the frail elderly; although efficacy is lower than in younger patients, the incidence of postoperative retention is also reduced.

Urinary frequency and nocturia. As the bladder ages, its functional capacity decreases and filling symptoms such as urgency and frequency become more prevalent. Nocturia is particularly common in the elderly and is discussed in Chapter 8. Bladder filling symptoms may be secondary to detrusor overactivity; however, intravesical pathologies such as tumors are more likely than in younger patients and further investigation with urine culture, cytology, urodynamic studies and cystoscopy may be required.

Voiding dysfunction. Poor detrusor contractility is common in the elderly and can impair voiding even in the absence of bladder outlet obstruction. Urinary retention may follow, which, if chronic, may be painless but can lead to overflow incontinence. It is also common for factors such as constipation, medication (such as antimuscarinics and α-adrenergic agonists) and bed rest to unmask subclinical voiding dysfunction and lead to retention.

Neurological problems can lead to voiding dysfunction. These include spinal cord compression resulting from a tumor or vertebral collapse, stroke, sensory loss and Parkinson's disease. Stroke may initially cause retention, which is replaced by neurogenic detrusor overactivity. Parkinson's disease results in voiding dysfunction, primarily as a result of detrusor overactivity, bradykinesia of the striated sphincter or poor detrusor contractility. Sensory loss is most commonly caused by diabetes; it may lead to progressive bladder distension, voiding dysfunction and acontractility, resulting in overflow incontinence.

Urinary retention. The aims of initial management are to stop any implicated factors such as medication and to rectify any reversible factors, such as prolapse in women. If this fails then the treatment of choice is self-catheterization. However, this may not be feasible for the reasons outlined above, and long-term suprapubic catheterization may be the only option (see pages 104–6).

Urinary tract infections are common in elderly women, occurring in up to 46% over the course of a year. This is normally the result of multiple factors, such as impaired immunology, voiding dysfunction and urinary stasis, genital atrophy from decreased estrogen, fecal incontinence and low fluid intake. There is also an increased likelihood of intravesical pathology. Investigation with flexible cystoscopy is recommended in the case of recurrent UTIs.

Treatment of UTIs in elderly women with no identifiable pathology is with low-dose vaginal estrogen and prophylactic antibiotics, as described in Chapter 7.

Polypharmacy (the use of multiple medications concurrently) is common in the elderly, and incontinence is frequently a result of medications prescribed for other conditions. Drugs can adversely affect bladder function in a number of ways, summarized in Table 10.1.

Pregnancy

Lower urinary tract symptoms are common during pregnancy, and childbirth is often cited as a cause for subsequent urinary, colorectal and genital dysfunction. The hormonal effects of pregnancy also can be responsible for other urinary tract pathology such as hydronephrosis and UTIs.

Bladder filling symptoms

Frequency. Between 45% and 90% of women will develop urinary frequency as pregnancy progresses. This is the result of increased renal blood flow, which increases urine production, and compression of the bladder by the enlarging uterus.

TABLE 10.1

Adverse effects of drugs on bladder function

Increased diuresis	• Diuretic medications and alcohol increase the rate of bladder filling and aggravate lower urinary tract symptoms
Decreased detrusor contractility	• Antimuscarinics, α-adrenergic agonists and calcium-channel blockers can decrease bladder contractility, and can precipitate urinary retention and subsequent overflow incontinence in a patient with poor intrinsic detrusor function
Alterations in urethral tone	• α-adrenoceptors may be responsible for the urethral sphincter tone; any medications that act as α-adrenergic agonists may therefore precipitate urinary retention, and antagonists may aggravate incontinence
	• β-adrenergic agonists, particularly β_2-agonists, and benzodiazepines can cause muscle relaxation and exacerbate urinary stress incontinence

Urgency is a common symptom in pregnancy, reported by up to 70% of women. It has been proposed that high progesterone levels may be the cause of detrusor overactivity in pregnancy, although urodynamic findings show detrusor overactivity in only approximately 25% of women who complain of urgency incontinence in pregnancy.

Antimuscarinic medication is contraindicated in pregnancy, so management is limited to bladder training, pelvic floor muscle exercises and restriction of caffeine intake.

Nocturia is common in pregnancy and is rarely pathological. It is caused by increased urine production and mobilization of dependent edema when the legs are elevated during sleep.

Urinary incontinence. Stress urinary incontinence in pregnancy is common – it has been reported in up to 85% of pregnant women. It is likely to be caused by pressure from the pregnant uterus, combined with relaxation of the pelvic ligaments and smooth musculature in response to the high levels of progesterone and other pregnancy hormones.

Prenatal stress incontinence usually resolves spontaneously after delivery, and the mainstay of treatment is pelvic floor muscle exercises (see Table 3.3, page 39). However, at least 25% of women will persist with incontinence post-delivery and these women will benefit from a structured and supervised pelvic floor muscle training program.

Intrapartum risk factors. A number of intrapartum events have been shown to contribute to postnatal urinary stress incontinence. Vaginal delivery, particularly in association with a prolonged second stage, assisted delivery, high birth weight and third-degree perineal tears can damage the pelvic floor innervation and increase pudendal nerve latency. Delivery with forceps appears to be associated with a higher incidence of stress incontinence than vacuum extraction and unassisted delivery.

While there is a widely held belief that Cesarean section protects against postpartum incontinence, the link is controversial and the evidence around it is conflicting. A prospective study of 1169 women undergoing elective Cesarean section showed that although the incidence of incontinence was reduced at 6 months postpartum, Cesarean section did not prevent incontinence.

It therefore seems likely that both pregnancy and any mode of delivery can cause pelvic floor dysfunction.

Voiding symptoms

During pregnancy one-third of women report hesitancy and an inability to empty their bladder completely. However, these symptoms are rarely associated with voiding disorders on urodynamic testing.

Urinary retention occurs occasionally, usually in association with entrapment of a retroverted uterus in the second trimester. Management involves bladder drainage and manual reduction of the uterus. If retroversion recurs, a pessary can be inserted temporarily to keep the uterus in the anteverted position, relieving the obstruction on the bladder neck.

Postnatal disorders. The most common cause of postnatal voiding disorders and urinary retention is the use of epidural and spinal anesthesia during labor and delivery. However, all women are at risk of urinary retention, and careful surveillance during and after delivery is important. Urinary retention requires prompt catheterization. It should be noted that many women have reduced bladder sensation after delivery, and urinary retention may not present with pain. Failure to recognize and manage postpartum urinary retention risks long-term bladder damage as a result of overdistension, denervation and atony of the detrusor muscle, which may require long-term catheterization.

Hydronephrosis is a common finding in pregnancy and is related to ureteral smooth muscle relaxation and the pressure of the enlarged uterus. It is more common on the right side. Hydronephrosis is largely asymptomatic and does not require treatment, and will resolve spontaneously on delivery.

If a woman presents with pain secondary to hydronephrosis, analgesia is usually all that is required. In the rare cases of renal impairment secondary to obstruction, ureteric stenting or percutaneous nephrostomy under radiological guidance is indicated.

Urinary tract infections. The smooth muscle relaxation associated with high levels of progesterone in pregnancy may predispose women to UTIs by affecting bladder emptying and ureteric drainage. UTIs are known to be associated with preterm delivery and low birth weight, so screening for infection and administering correct treatment are important.

Asymptomatic bacteriuria refers to the finding of more than 105 colony-forming units (CFU) per mL urine, which develops into pyelonephritis in 20–40% of pregnant women if left untreated, but only 1–2% if treated adequately.

Pregnant women should be screened for UTI at all antenatal visits; if a UTI has been treated, the patient should be followed up closely for signs of recurrence. If recurrent UTIs occur, then appropriate low-dose prophylactic antibiotics may be used until delivery.

Fistula-related incontinence

A fistula is an abnormal communication between two epithelialized structures. The urinary tract fistula most commonly responsible for urinary incontinence is the vesicovaginal fistula (VVF; Figure 10.1).

Etiology of VVF differs in various parts of the world. In developed countries, 75% of cases are iatrogenic, caused by injury to the bladder at the time of pelvic or gynecologic surgery. Obstetric trauma accounts for very few cases of VVF in developed countries, but is still a common cause in developing countries as a result of prolonged unsupervised labor. Other causes of VVF include pelvic malignancy, radiotherapy, trauma and gynecologic/urologic instrumentation.

Diagnosis. A woman with a VVF will commonly complain of continuous drainage of urine from the vagina, although small fistulas can present with intermittent urine leakage that is positional in nature. If the fistula is large, the patient may not void normally at all and may have continuous leakage of urine into the vagina.

A VVF that has occurred after surgery commonly presents upon removal of the urethral catheter or up to 3 weeks later with urinary drainage from the vagina. VVF caused by radiation therapy may present many months or even years after completion of radiotherapy.

It is important to distinguish VVF from other causes of urinary incontinence; investigations should include a full examination. If a fistula is suspected but is not identified on examination with a Sims'

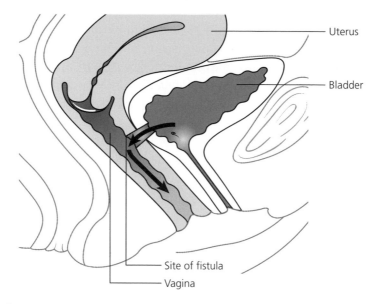

Figure 10.1 A vesicovaginal fistula.

speculum, further investigations will be needed to make the diagnosis. Even when the diagnosis can be made clinically, investigation may be needed to plan treatment.

Investigations

Examination under anesthesia may be required to determine the presence of a fistula. It is also important to assess the mobility of the tissues and the accessibility of a fistula for surgical repair.

Cystoscopy may also be carried out as part of this investigation. Although there is some debate as to the role of cystoscopy in the management of fistulas, it does enable the exact level of the fistula and its relation to the ureteric orifices and bladder neck to be assessed. In addition, a biopsy should be performed of the edge of any fistula that is related to radiotherapy or thought to be malignant.

Dye studies. The site of a fistula can be identified by instilling methylene blue dye into the bladder via a catheter, with the patient in the lithotomy position. The vagina is then inspected and the presence of fistulous communications noted. If urine continues to leak into the vagina despite a negative dye test, a ureteric fistula must be suspected.

Intravenous or CT urography (IVU/CTU) should be performed in all cases of suspected urinary tract fistula. Although IVU is not particularly sensitive in the diagnosis of VVF, knowledge of the upper urinary tracts may be important when considering treatment. Ureteric dilatation is commonly seen with ureteric fistulas; if it is found in association with a known VVF then a complex fistula should be suspected.

Retrograde pyelouretrography is useful to identify the exact site of a ureteric fistula or to definitely rule one out, and can be undertaken at the same time as therapeutic stenting of the ureter.

Treatment

Conservative management. The initial management of most urinary tract fistulas is generally conservative. VVFs may heal spontaneously with continuous bladder drainage with an indwelling catheter, over a period of 6–8 weeks, and a ureterovaginal fistula may resolve if the affected ureter is stented for 6–12 weeks. During the period of conservative management, the patient should be provided with incontinence pads and with barrier cream to protect the vulval and perineal skin, which is at risk of dermatitis as a result of prolonged contact with urine.

Surgical management. There is some debate as to the timing of surgical treatment of urinary tract fistulas. Early treatment is advocated by some because of the social and psychological benefits to women who are already distressed. However, fistulas may be associated with tissue inflammation and sloughing, and success rates are reduced if surgery is performed before this has resolved. It is therefore important not to be pressured by the patient into operating on a fistula too soon, as this may jeopardize the surgical outcome.

Fistulas can be repaired vaginally or abdominally; the principle of repair is the same for both routes. The fistula is identified and its tract excised. The layers are then closed. Success can be enhanced by interposition of healthy tissue between the bladder and vagina to create an additional layer to the repair. Tissues commonly used are omentum or a Martius graft of labial fat and bulbocavernosus muscle passed subcutaneously to cover the repair.

Key points – special considerations

- The prevalence of urinary tract symptoms increases with age, and urinary incontinence is a frequent cause of institutionalization of the elderly.
- Identification of the cause is more important in the elderly than in younger patients, as elderly patients are likely to have multiple coexisting symptoms and pathologies. Polypharmacy may be a contributory factor.
- Urinary tract infection (UTI) is common in elderly women. Treatment of persistent UTI is with low-dose vaginal estrogen and prophylactic antibiotics.
- Lower urinary tract problems are common in pregnancy and usually resolve after delivery.
- Vaginal delivery, especially associated with a long second stage of labor, forceps-assisted delivery and high birth weight, may damage the pelvic floor innervation and result in postnatal incontinence.
- UTIs are common in pregnancy and are associated with preterm delivery and low birth weight. Pregnant women should therefore be screened for UTIs at all antenatal visits, and UTIs treated accordingly.
- Vesicovaginal fistula (VVF), which results in vaginal leakage of urine, is the most common fistula to cause urinary incontinence.
- In developed countries, VVF may be caused by pelvic malignancy, radiotherapy, trauma and gynecologic/urologic instrumentation. Obstetric trauma during unsupervised labor is a common cause of VVF in developing countries.
- Dye studies and imaging are required to determine the site of a fistula.
- Many fistulas heal spontaneously over 6–12 weeks with conservative management such as bladder draining or ureteric stenting. Premature surgery is likely to be unsuccessful because of tissue inflammation and sloughing.

Key references

FitzGerald MP, Graziano S. Anatomic and functional changes of the lower urinary tract during pregnancy. *Urol Clin North Am* 2007;34:7–12.

Genadry R. A urogynecologist's view of the pelvic floor effects of vaginal delivery/cesarean section for the urologist. *Curr Urol Rep* 2006;7:376–83.

Ismail SI, Emery SJ. The prevalence of silent postpartum retention of urine in a heterogeneous cohort. *J Obstet Gynaecol* 2008;28:504–7.

Roush KM. Social implications of obstetric fistula: an integrative review. *J Midwifery Womens Health* 2009;54:e21–33.

Wagg AS, Cardozo L, Chapple C et al. Overactive bladder syndrome in older people. *BJU Int* 2007;99: 502–9.

Wall LL. Obstetric vesicovaginal fistula as an international public-health problem. *Lancet* 2006; 368:1201–9.

Useful resources

UK
Association for Continence
Advice
Tel: +44 (0)1506 811077
www.aca.uk.com

Bladder and Bowel Foundation
Helpline: 0845 345 0165
Tel: +44 (0)1536 533240
www.bladderandbowelfoundation.
org

**British Association of Urological
Surgeons**
Tel: +44 (0)20 7869 6950
www.baus.org.uk

**The Cystitis and Overactive
Bladder Foundation**
Tel: +44 (0)121 702 0820
www.cobfoundation.org

**Enuresis Resource and
Information Centre**
Helpline: 0845 370 8008
www.eric.org.uk

PromoCon
*(Product information, advice and
practical solutions for people with
continence difficulties)*
Helpline: 0161 607 8219
Tel: +44 (0)161 607 8200
www.promocon.co.uk

USA
American Academy of Family
Physicians
Toll-free: 1 800 274 2237
Tel: +1 913 906 6000
www.aafp.org

American Urological Association
Toll-free: 1 866 746 4282
Tel: +1 410 689 3700
www.auanet.org

**International Foundation for
Functional Gastrointestinal
Disorders**
Tel: +1 414 964 1799
www.iffgd.org
www.aboutincontinence.org

Interstitial Cystitis Association
www.ichelp.org

National Association For
Continence
Tel: +1 843 377 0900
www.nafc.org

National Kidney Foundation
Tel: +1 800 622 9010
www.kidney.org

Society of Urologic Nurses &
Associates
Toll-free: 1 888 827 7862
www.suna.org

Urology Channel
*(Comprehensive, physician-
monitored information about
urologic conditions)*
www.urologychannel.com

UroToday
(Comprehensive website about
urologic conditions)
www.urotoday.com

International
Campaign to End Fistula
www.endfistula.org

Canadian Paediatric Society
www.caringforkids.cps.ca/
growinglearning/Bedwetting.htm

Continence Foundation of
Australia
Toll-free: 1 800 33 00 66
Tel: +61 03 9347 2522
www.continence.org.au

European Association of Urology
Tel: +31 (0)26 389 0680
www.uroweb.org

International Continence Society
Tel: +44 (0)117 944 4881
www.icsoffice.org

Index

What the reviewers say:

www.fastfacts.com

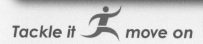

embarrassing problems.com

Tackle it move on

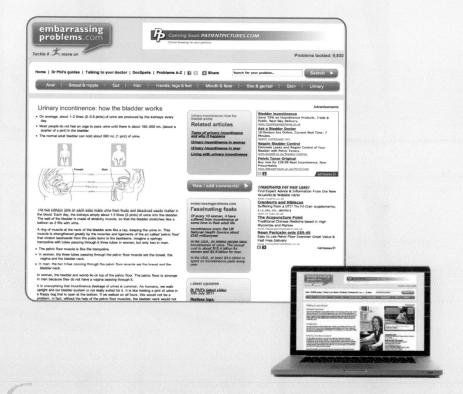

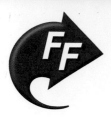
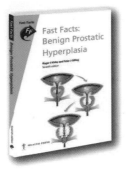
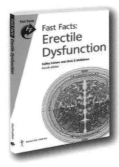
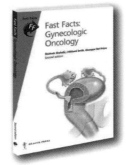
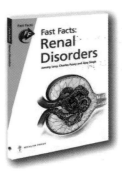
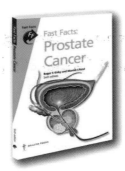
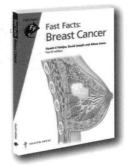
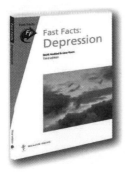
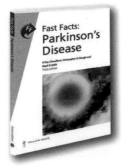
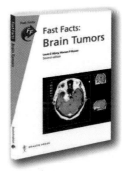